A Volume in The Laboratory Animal Pocket Reference Series

The Laboratory
CAT

The Laboratory Animal Pocket Reference Series

Editor-in-Chief
Mark A. Suckow, D.V.M.
Laboratory Animal Program
Purdue University
West Lafayette, IN

Advisory Board

B. Taylor Bennett, D.V.M., Ph.D.
Biologic Resources Laboratory
University of Illinois at Chicago
Chicago, IL

John Harkness, D.V.M., M.S., M.Ed.
College of Veterinary Medicine
Mississippi State University
Mississippi State, MS

Terrie Cunliffe-Beamer, D.V.M., M.S.
The Jackson Laboratory
Bar Harbor, ME

Roger P. Maickel, Ph.D.
Laboratory Animal Program
Purdue University
West Lafayette, IN

Published and Forthcoming Titles

The Laboratory Rabbit
The Laboratory Non-Human Primates
The Laboratory Mouse
The Laboratory Guinea Pig
The Laboratory Rat
The Laboratory Hamster and Gerbil
The Laboratory Cat
The Laboratory Small Ruminant

A Volume in The Laboratory Animal Pocket Reference Series

The Laboratory
CAT

Brent J. Martin, D.V.M.
Diplomat ACLAM
Director, Vivarium/Animal Resources
University of California
Santa Barbara, California

Editor-in-Chief
Mark A. Suckow, D.V.M.

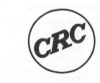

CRC PRESS

Boca Raton   London   New York   Washington, D.C.

Library of Congress Cataloging-in-Publication Data

Martin, Brent J.
   The laboratory cat/Brent J. Martin.
       p. cm. (The laboratory animal pocket reference series)
   Includes bibliographical references and index.
   ISBN 0-8493-2567-6
   1. Cats—research. 2. Biology—laboratory animals. I. Martin, Brent J.
   2. Biology—molecular. I. McLachlan, Alan. II. Title.
II. Title. III. Series.
BR749.H79G87   1997
616′.0149—dc20   97-25413

Visit the CRC Press Web site at www.crcpress.com

dedication

There are a number of people that I would like to mention and thank for their role in my life and this book. Dr. Daniel Ringler, my mentor and role model, has been instrumental in defining my professional career. Dr. Mark Suckow, a good friend and colleague, is regrettably greatly under appreciated for the impressive scientist that he is. I would like to thank my parents whose instillation of sound moral values and whose non-judgmental parenting style fostered independence that has made my success possible. I would like to thank my son, Sam, for the tremendous joy he brings into my life. I am continually amazed by what an impressive little person he is. Special thanks and ultimate dedication of this book go to my wife, Kathy, who has stuck by me through thick and thin.

preface

The use of laboratory animals continues to be an important part of biomedical research. Individuals performing such research are charged with broad responsibilities, including animal facility management, animal husbandry, regulatory compliance, and performance of technical procedures directly related to research projects. In this regard, this series of handbooks was developed to provide a quick reference source for investigators, technicians, and animal caretakers charged with the care and/or use of animals in research or teaching situations. These handbooks should be particularly valuable to those at small institutions or facilities lacking a large, well-organized animal resource unit and to those individuals who need to begin research programs using animals and beginning from scratch.

Volumes in this series have been developed for the mouse, the rat, the rabbit, the hamster and gerbil, the cat, the small ruminant, and the nonhuman primate. It is likely that as new procedures, techniques, and animal models are developed, additional volumes will be added to the series.

Information provided in this series has been extensively referenced. The user is thereby directed to sources of specific information for greater detail on topics beyond the scope of the series.

It is the ultimate hope of the editor, that the books in this series will facilitate biomedical research within the context of humane animal care and use.

This book is organized into six chapters: Important Biological Features (Chapter 1), Husbandry (Chapter 2), Management (Chapter 3), Veterinary Care (Chapter 4), Experimental Methodology (Chapter 5), and Resources (Chapter 6). Basic information and common procedures are presented in detail. Other information regarding alternative techniques, or details of procedures and methods which are beyond the scope of this book is referenced extensively so that the user is directed toward additional information without having to wade through a burdensome volume of detail here. In this sense, this book should be viewed as a basic reference source and not as an exhaustive review of the biology and use of the cat.

The final chapter, "Resources", provides the user with lists of possible sources and suppliers of additional information, cats, feed, sanitation supplies, cages, and research and veterinary supplies. The lists are not exhaustive and do not imply endorsement of listed suppliers over suppliers not listed. Rather, these lists are meant as a starting point for users to develop their own lists of preferred vendors of such items.

A final point to be considered is that all individuals performing procedures described in this handbook should be properly trained. The humane care and use of cats is improved by initial and continuing education of personnel and this will facilitate the overall success of programs using cats in research, teaching, or testing.

the author

Brent J. Martin is Director, Vivarium and Campus Veterinarian at the University of California in Santa Barbara, CA.

Dr. Martin earned the degree of Doctor of Veterinary Medicine from the Oregon State University in 1985 and completed a postdoctoral residency program in laboratory animal medicine at the University of Michigan in 1988. He is a Diplomate of the American College of Laboratory Animal Medicine.

Dr. Martin has responsibility for all veterinary and managerial operations at UCSB. He is the author 16 publications and abstracts covering a variety of aspects of laboratory animal science.

contents

1 IMPORTANT BIOLOGICAL FEATURES   **1**

Introduction   1
Origin of the Cat   1
Breeds   2
Behavior   3
Anatomical and Physiological Features   4
Normative Values   6

2 HUSBANDRY   **9**

Housing   9
Environmental Conditions   12
Environmental Enrichment   13
Nutrition   15
Sanitation   18
  Frequency   18
  Methods   19
  Quality Control   20
Transportation   21
Record Keeping   23
Breeding   26
  Reproductive Cycle   26
  Mating Behavior   26
  Pregnancy   27

3 MANAGEMENT   **29**

Regulatory Agencies and Compliance   29
Institutional Animal Care and Use Committee (IACUC)   31
Cat Quality   33

Sources   33
Quarantine and Condition   35
Occupational Health and Zoonotic Diseases   36

4 VETERINARY CARE   **41**
Basic Veterinary Supplies   41
Physical Examination   42
Common Clinical Problems   44
    Feline Urological Syndrome (FUS)   44
    Retroviral Diseases   45
    Abscesses   46
    Dermatophytosis (Ringworm)   46
    Ear Mites   47
    Intestinal Parasitism   47
    Fleas   47
    Respiratory Infections   47
    Feline Infectious Peritonitis (FIP)   48
    Enteric Diseases (Diarrhea)   49
    Metabolic Disorders   49
    Implant Problems   50
Treatment of Disease   50
    General Treatment of Dehydration   50
    General Treatment of Anorexia   52
    General Treatment of Open Skin Lesions 52
    Disease Prevention Through Sanitation 53
Anesthesia and Analgesia   53
    Definitions Commonly Used in Animal Anesthesia 54
    Choosing an Anesthesia Regimen   55
    Pre-Anesthesia Evaluation   57
    Pre-Anesthetic Medications   59
    Administering Anesthesia   59
    Monitoring Anesthesia   61
    Anesthesia Recovery   63
    Anesthesia Records   64
    Suggested Anesthesia Regimes   64
    Analgesia Dosages   66
Aseptic Surgery   66
    Postsurgical Management   67
Euthanasia   68

5 EXPERIMENTAL METHODOLOGY   71

Cats as Research Models   71
Handling   72
Handling Devices   77
Administering Medicines and Compounds   80
   Oral   80
   Parenteral   84
Urine Collection   91
Measuring Body Temperature   93
Endotracheal Intubation   93
Necropsy   94

6 RESOURCES   99

Organizations   99
Publications   101
Electronic Resources   103
Animal Sources   104
Feed   105
Equipment   105
   Sanitation   105
   Cages and Research and Veterinary Supplies   105
   Contact Information for Cages, Research, and
      Veterinary Supplies   106

BIBLIOGRAPHY   109

INDEX   129

important biological features

introduction

Cats have been used in research for many years. Investigators have tended to limit the use of cats to specialized research, and hence, the number of animals used has been small. The U.S. Department of Agriculture's figures show that 74,259 cats were used in research in 1974 and the use has consistently decreased since then. In 1995, 29,569 cats were used in research.[1] An adult male cat is called a **tom or stud** and an adult female cat is called a **queen**; however these terms are not widely used. An immature cat is called a **kitten**.

origin of the cat

The domestic cat, *Felis sylvestris catus*, is a member of the Family Felidae in the order Carnivora. The family contains close relatives such as the lynx and ocelot as well as more distantly related lions, tigers, and leopards. Cats are lithe and muscular predators with broad heads and short muzzles. With the exception of the cheetah, all cats have distinctly retractable claws.

Cats are believed to have been semi-domesticated from the Caffre wildcat, *Felis sylvestris libyca*.[2,3] The Caffre cat is a north African species living in the Nile River valley. Domestication appears not to have been a planned process, but rather, developed as a consequence of their proximity to the Egyptians.[4] This association with man probably developed circa 2500 B.C. as the cats hunted rodents feeding on the Egyptians' stores of grain.[3,5]

Cats achieved great stature in Egyptian culture: they were the objects of worship and their likenesses contributed to the images of gods. Other cultures in the Mediterranean apparently did not uniformly recognize cats as deities as they were widely traded throughout the region. Archeological findings suggest that cats were introduced to the British Isles by the Romans. From objects of worship in Egypt to loathsome tools of deviltry and witchcraft in the Middle Ages, cats nonetheless prevailed, spreading around the world by controlling the rodents that plagued the civilizations of man.[3]

breeds

With the dissemination of cats throughout the world came the development of a wide variety of breeds. Breeds are recognized groups of animals that are visibly recognizable as related. Some breeds represent a concentration of physical traits found in the general cat population, such as the Maine Coon and Russian Blue breeds. Other breeds represent unusual genetic variants maintained through selective breeding. Rare breeds such as the Scottish Fold and the American Curl demonstrate unusual ear configurations originating from genetic mutations.[3]

Some of the breed characteristics can reflect physical or biochemical features to be sought or avoided in research. The Maine Coon breed is a very large cat weighing 10 to 12 pounds, nearly twice the weight of most cats. Overall, cats tend to be fairly uniform in size and this large breed may have special utility in some specialized research. The Siamese and Manx breeds represent cats with genetic defects. Siamese cats have a defect in the tyrosinase gene which is instrumental in the characteristic coat color pattern.[3] This defect also causes disruption of the normal visual cross-over pattern of neural development making them unsuitable as a model for normal neural development.[6]

Siamese cats also demonstrate different cardioaccelerator responses than do other breeds.[7] Manx cats are distinctive in lacking a tail, a trait based upon an autosomal dominant genetic defect.[3] The breed characteristic is variable, but is a manifestation of neural tube developmental deficits and has been proposed as a spontaneous animal model for spina bifida research.[8]

While these specialized traits may be desirable or essential for specific research projects, cats with these traits are rare. Genetic traits among cats have been reviewed elsewhere.[9] Rare animals tend to be expensive and difficult to procure. In most cases, the specialized traits are not desirable for research and a standard cat is needed. The breed type that is most widely used in research is a medium-sized, short-haired cat, generally referred to as a domestic short hair or DSH.

behavior

While cats seem to have quite different personalities, some basic personality types such as confident and friendly vs. timid are consistently recognized. Interestingly, there is some evidence that basic personality has an hereditary basis, being influenced by paternal heritage.[10] A behavioral trait that is genetic is an attraction to catnip; approximately 50% of cats possess this trait.[11]

The social nature of cats is a subject of popular debate — they are frequently characterized as anti-social yet with ready examples to the contrary. This apparent conflict is partially reflected by strong individual variations between cats.[12] In studies of feral cats, it has been found that social behavior is rather restrained. Generally, feral cats are solitary and actively avoid each other. The vast majority of social behavior that occurs is between adults and juveniles.[12] Female cats tend to be amicable within familiar groups, however.[12] Social hierarchies develop in communally housed cats; this social interaction can be stressful. In contrast, cats readily adapt to solitary living.[11]

Cats communicate with each other through scent marking. Glands near the anus, perioral region, and feet are involved in marking as well as by urine.[12] Cats also communicate through visual cues which can be used by handlers to assess their attitude. These behavioral cues have been reviewed.[11] Two behaviors that handlers should watch for are repeated attempts to walk away from the researchers and a side-to-side twitching of the tail tip. Both behaviors signify that the cat is becoming irritated by the proceedings and may turn violent if care is not taken.

Without proper early **socialization**, cats, either specifically bred for research in large colonies or those from random sources, can be behaviorally undesirable. They may be excessively timid and fearful and they may be thoroughly intractable to handling. Use of asocial cats is extremely unpleasant for the facility and research staff and is apparently quite stressful for those cats.[10] Social relationships develop most readily within the first 2 months of age.[6] It is not known how much handling is optimal for socializing kittens, but it has been found that handling for 40 minutes per day is more effective than 15 minutes per day. Socialization by more than one person appears to make kittens more accepting to humans than if they are socialized by only one person.[10]

Surprisingly, the socialization of cats to human interaction apparently must be done as early as the second week of life with optimal effectiveness during the third week. This critical period is much earlier than that reported for dogs. Puppies are often socialized during weaning at 7 to 8 weeks of life. By weaning age, socializing kittens to humans can be done but its effectiveness is diminished.[10]

Particularly when considering avenues of augmenting the environment for enrichment purposes, it is essential to consider the predatory nature of cats. Play-type activities in cats tend to reflect **predatory behavior**.[6] Although hunting methods become modified by experience with prey-type, predatory behavior tends to be oriented around specialization for rodents.[13] Cats are attracted to and explore burrow-like areas such as cracks and crevices. Furthermore, they focus their attention by sound of movement and respond to rodent-sized objects moving in a straight line. Cats also key into object movement that is of appropriate speed for a rodent.[13]

anatomical and physiological features

Texts detailing the anatomy of cats are available.[14] The anatomic and physiologic features of cats are typical for their phylogenetic classification:

Chordata
  Vertebrata
    Mammalia
      Carnivora
        Fissipedia
          Feloidea
            Felidae
              Felis catus

Cats are characterized by a short, wide snout and large, forward-facing eyes. They have long, lithe bodies with their weight supported on their toes, called a digitigrade stance. Cats can supinate, or rotate their forepaws towards the medial plane, more so than most other animals. This being an adaptation for the capture of prey. The most unique anatomical feature of Felidae are their retractable claws. The tip of the last bone of the foot, called the third phalanx, has a sharp projection or "ungual process" that extends into the protective nail. The third phalanx and the enclosing claw are normally held in an extreme attitude where the bone lies to the side of the preceding phalanx. This is accomplished by a short ligament between the bones and has the effect of drawing the nail away from the ground and into a sheath of skin. Protrusion of the claws is an active process through contraction of muscles in the lower leg that pivots the nail forward and stretches the restraining ligament. Another uniquely feline feature is purring. The physiology of purring has been reviewed. in the literature.[15]

Generally, cat anatomy is quite similar to that of most terrestrial mammals and anatomical texts are readily available; however, a few features are worth mentioning:

1. Cats have five digits on the forelegs and four digits on the rear. Normally they support about 60% of their weight on their forelegs.

2. The male genitalia is small, furry, and set high near the anus, making determination of sex less readily apparent than in many other species. The penis has small spines on its surface and it is encased by a skin sheath called the prepuce. These structures are found directly ventral to the scrotum and are oriented towards the rear of the

cat rather than forward as in most animals. The teats are rudimentary in the male.

3. The feline skeleton encompasses 287 bones including a rudimentary collar bone. The vertebral column has 7 cervical, 13 thoracic, 7 lumbar, 3 sacral, and about 20 caudal vertebrae

4. The adult dental formula is $I_{3/3}$, $C_{1/1}$, $Pm_{3/2}$, $M_{1/1}$ and tooth wear can be used to roughly assess age.

5. Cats have a thin, but well-developed muscle layer in the subcutaneous regions of their entire body that can cause confusion to the inexperienced surgeon.

6. The spleen is comparatively large as in most carnivores. The jejunum and ileum encompass approximately 95% of the small intestine and they are reportedly of nearly equal length.

7. The large serosal fold called the greater omentum is a prominent feature of the abdominal cavity.

8. The cells of the convoluted and collecting tubules of the kidneys have an unusually high amount of fat that causes the kidneys to be pale, yellow-brown in color.

9. Cats have a well-developed third eyelid called the nictitating membrane. This lies in the inferior-medial area of the conjunctival sac and its movement across the eye is a passive process secondary to retraction of the eyeball into the orbit. The anatomy has been reported.[16]

normative values

Typical values for basic biological parameters (Table 1), clinical chemistries (Table 2), cerebrospinal fluid (Table 3), respiratory and cardiovascular function (Table 4), and hematology (Table 5) follow.

> **Note:** Normative values can vary significantly between clinical laboratories, breeds, ages, and sexes and the following tables reflect general guidelines that should be a basis for development of facility-specific tables.

TABLE 1. BASIC BIOLOGICAL PARAMETERS OF THE CAT

Parameter	Typical values	Reference(s)
Diploid chromosome number	38	17
Life span (years)	9–14	17, 18
Body weight (kg)	2.5–3.5	17
Body temperature (°C)	38.0–39.5	17, 18
Metabolic energy requirement (Kcal/kg/day)	70	19
Food intake (g/day)	240	18
Water intake (ml/day)	200–300	18
Upper GI transit time (hours)	2–3	20
Urine volume (ml/kg/day)	22–30	17, 21
Urine specific gravity	1.018–1.050	17, 21
Urine pH	5.5–8.5	17, 22

TABLE 2. CLINICAL CHEMISTRY VALUES OF THE CAT

Parameter	Typical value	Reference(s)
Total Protein (g/dl)	5.4–7.3	21
Globulin (g/dl)	2.6–5.1	21
Albumin (g/dl)	2.1–3.3	21
Amylase (IU/L)	700–1800	23
Alkaline phosphatase (IU/L)	2–7	21
LDH (IU/L)	16–69	21
Aspartate aminotransferase (SGOT) (IU/L)	15–35	23
Creatinine kinase (IU/L)	100–850	23
ALT (SGPT) (IU/L)	1.7–14	21
Blood urea nitrogen (mg/dl)	15–33	23
Glucose (mg/dl)	70–110	21
Sodium (meq/L)	147–156	21
Chloride (meq/L)	111–128	23
Potassium (meq/L)	4.0–4.5	21
Calcium (mg/dl)	9.1–12.3	23
Total Bilirubin (mg/dl)	0.15–0.20	21
Corticotropin (ng/L)	59–87	24
Alpha-melanocyte stimulating hormone (ng/L)	117–141	24
Cortisol (nmol/L)	71–103	24

TABLE 3.   CEREBROSPINAL FLUID VALUES OF THE CAT

Parameter	Typical value	Reference(s)
Cells (cells/mm^3)	0–5	21
Pressure (mm H$_2$0)	<100	25
Protein (mg/dl)	0–20	25
Specific gravity	1.005–1.007	21

TABLE 4.   VALUES FOR CARDIOVASCULAR AND RESPIRATORY FUNCTION OF THE CAT

Parameter	Typical value	Reference(s)
Respiratory rate (breaths/min)	20–40	17, 18
Heart rate (beats/min)	110–140	17
Tidal volume (ml/kg)	20–42	17
pO$_2$ (mm Hg)	31–49	23
pCO$_2$ (mm Hg)	35–49	23
HCO$_3^-$ (mEq/L)	18–22	23
Arterial systolic pressure (mm Hg)	120	17, 18
Arterial diastolic pressure (mm Hg)	75	17, 18
Arterial blood pH	7.24–7.40	17, 18

TABLE 5.   HEMATOLOGICAL VALUES OF THE CAT

Parameter	Typical value	Reference(s)
Packed cell volume (%)	30–45	8, 17
Red blood cells (10^6/ul)	5.0–10.0	17
Erythrocyte lifespan (days)	36.3–66.1	26
White blood cells (10^3/ul)	5.5–19.5	17
Hemoglobin (g/dl)	8–15	17, 27
Neutrophils (10^3/ul)	3–13	23
Lymphocytes (10^3/ul)	1.2–9	23
Eosinophils (10^3/ul)	0–1.2	23
Basophils (10^3/ul)	rare	17
Monocytes (10^3/ul)	0–0.7	23
Platelets (10^5/ul)	3–7	17
Reticulocytes (%)	0–1	17
MCV (fl)	82–92	27
MCHC (%)	31–35	27
MCH (pg)	13–17	27
Blood volume (ml/kg)	47.3–66.7	17, 27
Plasma volume (ml/kg)	34.6–52.0	17

2

husbandry

housing

A variety of caging options are available, from stainless steel cages large enough for one cat to open animal rooms.

> **Note:** The Standards of the Animal Welfare Act must be considered foremost when developing housing accomodations for cats.

The Animal Welfare Act has both general and specific requirements. The cage immediately surrounding the cat is called the primary enclosure. In general, the primary enclosure must be soundly constructed and well maintained. It must be constructed of materials that can be sanitized or replaced when worn or soiled. It must not have sharp projections that may cause injury. The cages should be routinely examined for broken welds and loose wires that develop through use. The cages must keep the animals in and other animals out. They must keep the animals clean and dry and provide ready access to food and water. If the primary enclosures are not located indoors, they must protect the animals from extremes in weather and provide sufficient shade for all the animals in the enclosure.

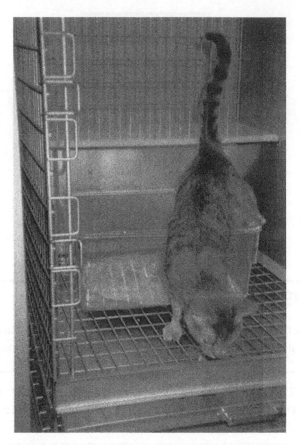

FIG. 1.   Primary enclosure for an individually housed cat. The front wall of the cage opens and has been swung out of the photograph. The white, plastic resting surface and the litter box are clearly visible.

Cat cages are frequently constructed with wire or mesh floors (Figure 1). The holes through the floor must be sufficiently small that the animals' legs cannot pass through them. The material and its construction must be such that legs and feet are not injured. All cages that have wire floors must supply a solid resting surface. Furthermore, there must be sufficient resting surfaces for all animals in the enclosure to recline at the same time. The resting surface must be elevated above the floor level. Cats prefer to use a litter box for defecation and urination and one should be supplied. Care must be taken in choosing non-toxic absorbent litter material.[28]

- The primary enclosure must permit the cats to move about freely and adopt a variety of body positions, such as standing, sitting, and lying down.

- The cage must have at least 24 inches of interior height from floor to ceiling. Cats weighing 8.8 pounds or less must have at least 3.0 square feet of floor space and heavier cats must have at least 4.0 square feet.

- Items in the enclosure, such as food and water pans that the animal cannot comfortably get under, must not be included in the floor space calculations.

- If a litter box is supplied, it can be counted as available floor space if it is properly cleaned and sanitized.

- The primary enclosure must have additional available space in the case of a mother with nursing litter.

Cats can be housed in a variety of ways. To a large extent, the options need to be weighed in relation to the research needs. Cats may be housed individually, in pairs or in groups (Figure 2).

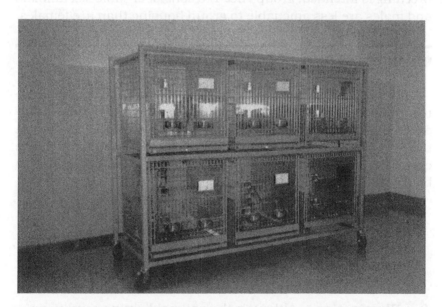

Fig. 2. Rack containing six cages. Construction materials are stainless steel except for the resting surface and litter box. Food and water bowls are attached to the cage fronts.

While multiple animals per cage can supply environmental enrichment, it also may represent social stress[11] and an infection control risk.[29] Experimental implants and surgery sites may also be disturbed by cage mates in multiple cat housing. Many cats, especially young females, can be successfully group housed; however, cats' social behaviors are not uniformly supportive of group housing. Social conflicts between animals can lead to injuries and distress. When cats are grouped, a number a things need to be considered. Groups should be established in a way that it is likely that the group can stay together. Separation of animals from the group and the repeated introduction of animals into a group causes continual stress. This increases the likelihood of conflict between the animals. Stress also has a wide physiological impact that can affect research results. When small groups of animals are going to be housed together, they should be introduced into the new cage space as a group. If one or two animals have previously been occupying the space, they may defend it as their own territory if new animals are introduced. This may be less of a problem in larger groups. Unless breeding is intended, groups need to consist of same sex animals and males are less amenable to group housing than are females.

environmental conditions

The foremost purpose of the laboratory animal facility is to maintain a controlled and stable environment such that influences other than the experiment are minimized. Variability in their surroundings may cause physiological adjustments in the cats that can effect experimental data. Important conditions to be controlled include:

1. **Temperature.** Cats tolerate a fairly wide range of ambient temperatures; however, temperature adaptations take time and involve physiological changes that can influence research. Temperatures should be stable within a few degrees and the fall in the range of 64°F to 84°F.

2. **Illumination.** Although the optimal lighting conditions for cats are unknown, common practice employs a 12 or 14 hour light to a 12 or 10 hour dark cycle. For breeding

colonies, the 12:12 cycle has been shown to be optimal.[30] Light should be sufficient to allow daily observation of cats within their cages.

3. **Ventilation.** Ventilation is important to maintain stability of gaseous and particulate contaminants and to dilute and remove heat and humidity generated by the animals. The ventilation must be well distributed throughout the room to effectively maintain the air quality and to minimize drafts. Ventilation rates of 10 to 15 room changes per hour are commonly employed for cat rooms.[31] Recirculation of room air is not advisable.

4. **Humidity.** Relative humidity is difficult to closely control. Recommended values for relative humidity are 30% to 70%.[31]

5. **Noise.** Cats may be startled by sudden, sharp noises. Personnel should exercise care to minimize noise in the presence of cats and facilities should be designed with due consideration for noise. Cat quarters should be shielded from noisy species such as dogs, swine, and nonhuman primates.

environmental enrichment

Increasingly, facilities are considering the **psychological impact** of the research environment on research animals. The impact of the environment has not been elucidated but elements for enrichment have been proposed based on the information currently available.[32] Some cats respond well to group housing that permits a variable and stimulating environment. In group housing situations, the area must have elevated resting boards that supply sufficient space for every cat in the enclosure. This is not only necessary to meet the welfare needs of the cats but it is also legally required by the Animal Welfare Act.[33] In practice, the resting areas should exceed this minimum as cats seek out solitary opportunities even in group housing situations. It has been reported that cats prefer soft resting areas constructed of insulating material over hard, conductive construction.[34] This is intuitive as well; but, use of towels and other soft bedding material must be weighed against considerations of sanitation. While making arrangements for rotating and cleaning bedding material are not insurmountable problems, supplying these materials is also not essential.

Small **play toys** for cats are readily available through veterinary supply houses and even pet and department stores. Cats do not particularly favor toys for chewing rather choosing devices that supply motion and sound through which their predatory behaviors can be stimulated.

Care and consideration must be made regarding the use of scented toys. **Catnip** scented toys are available. Catnip has been shown to elicit pleasure responses in cats.[11] Catnip originates from the plant, *Nepeta cataria* of the mint family. Chemical modification of behavior by use of catnip may represent an undesirable research variable. Catnip has biochemical similarities to marijuana and other psychedelic drugs.[11] The cost-benefit balance of use can only be assessed in context of the individual institution's research.

Cage complexities and resting areas may be wood or carpet tubes, boxes and poles that are disposed of when soiled and worn. Other institutions have had experience using standard laboratory plastic and steel carts and shelves that are very readily cleaned.

Solitary housing can be highly successful and it is preferred by some cats.[11] Depending on the individual cat's personality, it can be essential. Visual and olfactory contact is desirable. A resting board is essential. Toys may be supplied on the floor of the cage and can be suspended from the cage roof to add to the stimulation of the environment. A litter box must be supplied according to the Animal Welfare Act; however, a litter box and the litter itself appear to be important enrichment devices for cats and should always be supplied for this reason, as well.

Significant considerations with **group housing** are the probability of disease transmission, fighting and pregnancy.

- Disease transmission may be a lesser concern with specific pathogen-free cats than with random source animals.

- Group housed animals must be monitored to assure that animals are not injured by fighting. Males are less apt to be compatible than are females.

- Obviously, grouped animals must be of the same sex to avoid pregnancy unless other measures are taken to control reproduction.[35]

---

nutrition

Cats are **strict carnivores**, naturally eating a diet composed of more meat than dogs. Cats have fewer molar teeth, a smaller cecum, poor excretion systems for absorbed plant products and lower digestive efficiency than the dog, supporting the requirement for a strictly carnivorous diet.[36] Adaptation to the carnivorous diet has lead to a number of unique nutritional requirements. Since prey items readily supply arachidonate, taurine, arginine, niacin, and vitamin A, nutritional requirements for these have developed.[37] Information on cat nutrition is presented in greater detail elsewhere.[37]

While the carnivorous diet of cats is well established, meat alone is not nutritionally complete. This is particularly relevant to the minerals, calcium and phosphorous.[37] Cats should be fed a commercially prepared diet labeled as nutritionally complete for all stages of life (e.g., pregnancy, lactation, growth, and maintenance). Diets of this type are readily available. Complete diets prepared for the research environment should be used as they are formulated to minimize dietary variability.

If research protocols involve foods other than the standard diet, consideration must be given to the peculiarities of cats. They are intolerant of high carbohydrate diets.[36] They select against diets containing saccharin, cyclomate, and casein[38] and are not attracted to the taste of sucrose (table sugar).[36] They are sensitive to taste changes. Cats have a tendency to prefer foods experienced early in life.[38,39] It is generally wise to slowly introduce changes in diet by mixing increasing percentages of the new food into the diet.

Amount of feed. The recommended amount to be fed varies with the individual diet and cat. Naturally, cats eat numerous small meals scattered throughout the 24 hour day.[36,38] Generally, both immature and adult cats can be fed *ad libitum*. As a general guideline, adult cats will consume an average of 71 kcal per kg body weight.[38]

This may represent about 70 grams of dry or 190 grams of canned cat food per day.[40]

Presentation of feed. Feed is normally offered to cats in a bowl attached to the cage. It is important to offer the feed in such a way that contamination by urine or feces does not occur. Cats should be given fresh food each day as food odor is important to cat feeding.

Basic analysis. A typical dry cat food will contain approximately 31% protein, 11% fat, and 43% carbohydrate.

Taurine. Cats have a unique dietary requirement for the amino acid taurine. This is due to both a low taurine production in the liver secondary to low cysteine sulphinic acid decarboxylase enzyme activity and to a high taurine loss, since taurine is an obligatory conjugator of bile salts in the cat.[36,37] Deficiency of taurine causes degeneration of the retina and has been associated with cardiomyopathy.[41,42] Diets supplying taurine at 400 mg/kg diet (500 mg/kg diet for reproduction) are adequate.[37]

Vitamin A. Cats lack the dioxygenase enzyme required for the utilization of carotene as a source of vitamin A.[36] Therefore, vitamin A must be added to the diet at 1 mg retinol/kg diet (1.8 mg retinol/kg diet for reproduction).[37]

Thiamine. Cats have a high dietary requirement for thiamine, being approximately 4 times higher than the requirement for dogs. Thiamine deficiency has been seen in colony cats.[43,44] Deficiency may cause a loss of balance and convulsions. Five mg thiamine/kg diet is recommended.

Niacin. While cats possess a functional enzyme system for niacin production, an intermediate metabolite is utilized so rapidly that sufficient quantities of niacin are not produced. Therefore, it must be supplied in the diet at 40 mg/kg diet.

Storage of feed. In general, commercial pelleted cat feed will retain acceptable nutritive levels for approximately

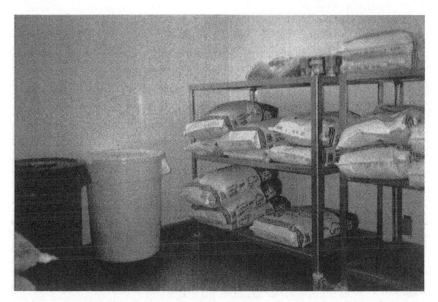

FIG. 3. Food and bedding storage area. The stocked feed bags on movable carts with milling dates clearly visible are set away from the wall for easy cleaning. The plastic barrels contain opened feed bags.

180 days after milling (Figure 3). For this reason, most reputable feed suppliers indicate the date of milling on the outside of feed packages. If the date is encoded, one may need to contact the feed supplier for code interpretation. Feed should be used no later than 180 days after the milling date.

Feed should be stored in a room which is neither excessively hot nor humid. Storage should be separate from storage of potentially hazardous substances such as insecticides or chemicals used for cleaning and disinfection. In addition, feed should be stored off the floor and away from the wall in order to facilitate sanitation. Open bags of feed should be stored in containers with tightly fitted lids, to minimize vermin contamination. Storage procedures should facilitate display of specific information regarding the date of milling or the expiration date of the feed. Spilled feed should be promptly cleaned up and discarded.

Water.   Cats should be provided a constant source of fresh, clean, potable water. Water can be provided by a bowl placed in the cage. Most commercially available cat cages have spaces for bowls that keeps them from being tipped over. Water intake can vary tremendously depending on individual cat preference and diet. On average, cats consume nearly twice as much water when fed a canned, wet diet than when fed a dry pelleted ration (when the water in the food is calculated into the formula).[38,45,46] This is important when considering management of feline urolithiasis (see diseases).

sanitation

Sanitation refers to the procedures and schedules for cleaning. All materials, surfaces and equipment must be considered when developing the sanitation program as soilage, even when undetectable visually, can provide substrate for microorganisms and harborage for vermin. To achieve this objective, issues such as frequency and methods of sanitation must be considered.

Frequency

Frequency of cage and room sanitation may depend upon factors including the number of animals per room and the types of cages used. Individual animals may require more cleaning and care efforts than is typical for cats in general. As a general guideline, the following schedule would be typical for cat husbandry:

- **Daily** — the litter boxes are removed and cleaned, feces and urine are spot cleaned from the cages and drop pans as necessary, feed bowls are removed and cleaned if canned cat food is used.

- **Two or three times per week** — drop pans, food bowls and water bowls are removed and cleaned, the animal room floor is swept or hosed.

- **Weekly** — cats are transferred to clean, disinfected cages (although some facilities opt to change cages biweekly).

- **Every 2 months** — the animal room walls, floor, and ceiling and the fixtures in the room are thoroughly cleaned and disinfected.

Methods

Both the caging and equipment that the cats directly contact and the surrounding rooms must be regularly sanitized. Sanitation involves removal of grossly visible debris such as hair and feces. It also involves removal of surface films of oil and dirt that may not be obviously seen. This complete **cleaning** process is necessary for effective disinfection. **Disinfection** refers to the reduction or elimination of harmful microorganisms. Disinfection cannot be effectively accomplished on porous, cracked, and rough surfaces nor on surfaces that are covered with dirt that shields the microorganisms from the disinfecting process.

surface cleaning

Grossly visible debris is generally washed off with running water. Brushing and rinsing with water may be sufficient for cleaning; however, detergents are usually used to loosen or dissolve debris and to lift oils and organics that often coat animal cages. Individuals performing these procedures should wear protective equipment to minimize the risk of chemical or thermal injury to the skin, eyes, and nasal passages. In addition, hearing protection is advisable due to the intensity of noise which may be generated by cage-washing operations.

disinfection

A variety of disinfectant chemicals are available from a number of vendors. The products used should be specifically formulated for the laboratory animal environment. These chemicals often have detergent properties and their use accomplishes both cleaning and disinfection. Any application of chemical to cages or equipment should be followed by thorough rinsing with water to minimize exposure of the animals to potentially harmful chemicals. Disinfection may also be accomplished with hot water. Typically, water at temperatures near 180°F is used for this step, although procedures using water at lower temperatures with longer sanitation times have been shown to be similarly effective.[47]

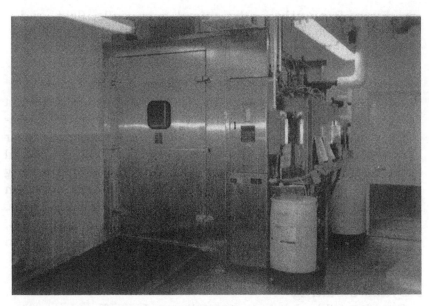

Fig. 4. Mechanical cage washing equipment for thorough sanitation.

> **Note:**   Personnel should wear protective equipment such as protective gloves, aprons, and safety goggles when handling chemicals used for sanitation.

Movable equipment may be effectively sanitized manually;[48] however, the use of automatic cage washers are more efficient and reproducible (Figure 4). The animal rooms and fixed equipment must be sanitized manually. The process of cleaning and disinfection is the same as for the cages. The chemical vendors can supply devices for cleaning and application of disinfectants.

> **Note:**   Animals should be removed from rooms or protected in such a way that they do not become wet nor exposed to chemicals during cleaning.

Quality Control
It is important that the sanitation effectiveness be monitored. On a daily basis, visual inspection and noticing odors is an

important test for overall efficacy. A more objective program for monitoring should also be put into place. Several methods may be employed in this regard:

sanitation temperature

Test tapes are available that will undergo a color change when exposed to temperatures consistent with disinfection. The strips of tape are applied to the cages prior to being washed in a mechanical cage washer. Monitoring with temperature tape is often performed weekly but may be done more frequently. Used tape samples can be maintained in a log as a record of acceptable cage wash temperature.

microbiologic monitoring

Since a major objective of sanitation is removal of microorganisms and the dirt that shield them, the best assay for sanitation efficacy involves bacterial culture of equipment and room surfaces. Surfaces which might be tested include animal room surfaces, cages, cage racks, water bottles, sipper tubes, feeders, and any other equipment that undergoes sanitation. Swabs of such surfaces may be cultured or Rodac plates can be gently touched against cage and room surfaces and incubated. Moderate bacterial growth indicates weakness in the disinfection process. Gram negative, rod-shaped organisms are the hallmark of fecal contamination and necessitates evaluation of the procedures.

---

transportation

Typically, cats are transported to the research facility and the shipping arrangements are made by the animal vendor. Research cats are frequently of defined infectious disease status; yet they may be exposed to "common" cats during transportation. Care must be taken to protect the cats from exposure to disease during shipping. Vaccination of the cats and applying filter paper over the ventilation openings in the containers are often done to help protect the cats.

Transportation of cats is intricately regulated. The research facility and the shipper must assure that the shipping and documentation fully complies with the regulations, primarily those of the Animal Welfare Act[33] in the U.S.A. For interstate shipments, specifications of the destination state may need to be met, as well. Intermediate carriers also have detailed requirements that they must adhere to and it is important to properly prepare shipped animals and their accompanying documentation to meet these regulations .[33] These regulations are critically important and complicated.

> **Note:** The Animal Welfare Act regulations should be consulted any time cats are shipped.

Briefly, important aspects of transportation include records, the shipping container, provision of food and water during transit, observation of cats during transit, and environmental factors.

Records. Commercially transported cats must be accompanied by a health certificate signed by a licensed veterinarian. The health certificate must be signed within 10 days of travel and must indicate that the cat appeared free of problems that would endanger the animal or other humans (see Part 2, Subpart C, 2.38, (h)) . An additional certificate must indicate who is sending the animals and the USDA assigned identification for each animals (see Part 3, Subpart A, 3.13, e). A signed and dated certification of temperature acclimation must be included by a licensed veterinarian (see Part 3, Subpart A, 3.13, (e)). Shipping documents must include feeding and watering instructions (see Part 3, Subpart A, 3.13, (c))

Shipping container (see Part 3, Subpart A, 3.14). The shipping container must securely and safely contain the animal. It should be constructed of material durable enough to securely contain the cat and withstand damage that could result in injury. It must indicate which side should face up and that it contains "Live Animals". Sufficient space should be provided to allow the cat to make normal postural adjustments and it should be designed to protect the cat from feces and urine. Containers should be designed to allow adequate ventilation of the container; the ventilation requirements are detailed. One cat per container is permitted for air travel and 4 compatible cats per container are permitted for ground transportation.

Food and water. The need to provide food and water during transportation depends upon the length of time and conditions of shipping. The Regulations of the Animal Welfare Act state that food and water must be provided within 4 hours of delivery to a commercial carrier (see Part 3, Subpart A, 3.13, (c)). Feeding and watering instructions must accompany the animals. At a minimum, cats must be supplied with water at least twice a day for at least 1 hour each time and they must be fed at least once a day (see Part 3, Subpart A, 3.16). Food and water receptacles must be secured inside the shipping containers for this purpose.

Observation. Frequent observation during transportation is recommended. The Regulations of the Animal Welfare Act require observation every four hours except during air shipment when it is not possible to do so (see Part 3, Subpart A, 3.17). Adequacy of ventilation, ambient temperature, and general condition of the cats should all be assured during observation. Any factors resulting in stress to the animal should be corrected as soon as possible. Animals developing health problems should receive prompt veterinary care.

Environment. Maintaining the environment that surrounds the cats during shipment is of great importance. The ventilation system should provide fresh air with minimal drafts. Extremes of temperature should be avoided. Cats should not be exposed to temperatures about 85 °F for more than 4 hours nor temperatures below 45 °F for periods greater than 45 minutes.

record keeping

Records are required for a variety of reasons. The animal facility husbandry can influence the research and hence the husbandry must be standardized. Records are instrumental in assuring that the husbandry is done in a routine and thorough manner. Several groups of users interact with the research cat and records help maintain continuity and communication between the husbandry staff, the veterinary care givers and the researchers. Specific records are also required by the regulations of the Animal Welfare Act. Because cats are a species of political concern, the USDA field inspectors show a particular interest in cat records.

In daily practice, records should be maintained such that they are easily accessible and understood by the users. However, records must be protected from water and animal damage and from misplacement. Plastic file boxes available at most office supply stores are excellent for protecting records in the animal facility environment. Plastic overlays and laminating are also often used for protection.

A number of records are specifically required by the regulations. It is very important that these be collected and maintained.

USDA Records. All cats must be uniquely identified in a USDA approved manner. This identification must be traceable from the time of acquisition until 3 years after disposal (the tag itself must be maintained for 1 year). The identification must be by tag or tattoo and include the letters "USDA", numbers identifying the facility and numbers identifying the specific animal.

Cats acquired, including those born in the facility, must have acquisition records. The records must identify the name and address of the supplier, their USDA registration or license number, the date of acquisition, the animal's USDA identification number, a complete description of that specific cat and any other identifying number applied to that cat.

There must be a record of disposal for all cats relinquished live from the research facility. These records include name and address of new holder, date of disposal, method of disposal, and a copy of the acquisition records.

Note: An annual report of research use must be filed with the USDA before December 1 each year detailing cat use during the previous federal fiscal year.

Other Identification. In addition to the strict identification records of the regulators, it is imperative to maintain cat identity during the research so that the results are properly applied to the treatment. Cage cards are routinely used for identification purposes. In addition to recording the USDA identification number, many facilities use a cage card to record information critical to the operation. This may include the investigator's name, the IACUC protocol number, the dates of acquisition and birth, the account number being recharged and the animal source. Cage cards are cheap and convenient; however, they are quite susceptible to destruction. Implantable microchip transponders called PIT (passive integrated transponder) tags can be a reliable way of identifying cats. These are 1 cm long glass vials containing a microchip that are implanted in the subcutaneous space. They respond with a unique identifying number when scanned by their reader.

Health Records. Adequate veterinary care requires an animal history when problems develop. Health records need to be generated for each cat as they enter the facility. This record should include pertinent health information from the supplier and records of on-going preventative health care, such as physical exams, treatments, and vaccinations. Additionally, records of experimental manipulations need to be recorded. Records maintained during and after surgery are particularly necessary. This information is necessary so that the veterinarian investigating a health problem can formulate a diagnostic care plan.

Census Records. Information concerning the number of animals in individual rooms and the overall facility is helpful in planning the daily work load. Census information maintained on a room card on the outside door and logged into a permanent record is often useful.

Work Records. Records of routine husbandry tasks carried out in animal rooms should be maintained. Basic relevant information includes food and water provision and intake, changing of cages and cage rack, temperature, date and time of day when the animals are checked, and initials of the individual logging the information.

breeding

It is rarely cost effective to breed and raise cats for research within a facility due to the low-reproductive output and their relatively slow rate of maturation. However, cats are sometimes used in developmental research where breeding may be necessary for experimental reasons.

Reproductive Cycle

Reproduction in cats has been extensively reviewed elsewhere.[49,50]

- **Puberty** Puberty in cats is quite variable generally occurring after attaining 2.5 kgs body weight.[50]

- **Estrus** Under natural light conditions, cats are seasonally polyestrus with females cycling winter through summer[49,50] but they will breed year around under controlled lighting.[49,51] The estrous cycle is roughly 2 to 3 weeks in length[49,52] but it is not as rigidly defined as in many species.[50] Both too long and too short of daylight length will adversely affect the estrous cycle with 14L:10D being preferred.[53] The estrus period is approximately 6 days long.[49,50]

- **Ovulation** Cats do not generally ovulate unless copulation has occurred. However, some cats will ovulate without copulation or genital stimulation[52] and ovulation can be hormonally induced.[54,55] Ovulation can be detected through measurements of progesterone in serum[52]; measurements of fecal progesterone may also be useful.[56]

Mating Behavior

Females tend to rub their head and neck against objects and roll on the floor when receptive. A breeding stance with pelvis raised above the crouched body and hindlegs trending can be readily elicited during estrus. A small amount of white fluid discharge from the vagina is also sometimes present during estrus. These behavioral signs of estrus are often present during the 1 to 2 day proestrus phase of the cycle when the females are not receptive to coitus. A tendency for queens to have synchronized estrus has been noted in colony settings.[57] Cats frequently breed multiple times but ovulation is most apt to be induced by a single copulation on the third day of estrus.[50] The intended stud often will not breed a female if he is not in his own territory; hence it is important to take the female to the male's cage.[49] The copulating male often bites the dorsal neck of the female and the female vocalizes. The queen will mate with multiple males if multiple males are available.[57] Ovulation is variable often requiring multiple mating to occur and the timing of ovulation is imprecise.[49,50] Infertile matings are followed by a pseudopregnancy period of 35 to 40 days.[58]

Pregnancy

- **Gestation** Gestation length is approximately 65 days long but it is very variable. Colonies have reported gestation lengths from 52 to 74 days[50,59] and gestation length differences related to genetic sublines have been documented.[59]

- **Pregnancy detection** The standard method for pregnancy detection is by abdominal palpation. Experienced palpators can identify fetuses between 15 and 35 days of gestation.[58] Skeletons begin to ossify at approximately 43 days allowing the use of X-ray imagery.[58] Fetal skulls can also often be palpated late in pregnancy. Fetal heart beats can be used for confirmation of pregnancy by 22 days after copulation.[60] Pregnant queens demonstrate a nearly linear increase in body weight gain and in food consumption throughout pregnancy ultimately gaining approximately 30% of their prepregnancy weight.[61] This suggests that early pregnancy diagnosis may be possible by detecting a 10% body weight increase by the 4th week following mating.[61]

- **Litters** Pregnancy failure can be related to current and past taurine deficiencies.[62] Litter size varies between one and five kittens and has been found to be highly correlated with prepregnancy body weight.[61] Litter size and litters per queen may be responsive to dietary changes.[63] *In vitro* fertilization techniques have been successful.[64,65] Problems at parturition are uncommon in most cat colonies but they are breed related.[66]

*   **Kittens** Kittens can be hand-raised with commercially available milk replacer.[67] Kittens are typically weaned at 7 to 8 weeks but under feral conditions, they tend to be weaned earlier (4 to 7 weeks).[68]

Table 6 indicates normal reproductive indices.

TABLE 6.   REPRODUCTIVE SYSTEM VALUES OF THE CAT

Parameter	Typical value	Reference(s)
Puberty, female (months)	6–10	49,50
Puberty, male (months)	8–12	49
Estrus cycle (days)	14–21	49, 52
Implantation (days post-coitus)	12–13	50
Gestation length (days)	58–67	17, 50, 59
Litter size (kittens)	3–6	17, 50, 69
Birth weight (g)	85–120	17, 50, 59

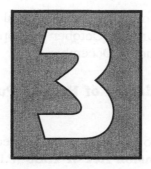

management

---

regulatory agencies and compliance

Specific regulatory agencies and requirements may vary with locale; however, in the United States the following are the primary organizations with regulatory oversight or accreditation responsibilities for programs of research, teaching, or testing:

The United States Department of Agriculture (USDA)

- Oversight responsibility is described in the **Animal Welfare Act** (P.L. 91-579, 94-279, 99-198).[70] The Animal Welfare Act is often abbreviated as AWA and the term is frequently used synonymously with the regulations promulgated under the AWA.

- Specific standards or requirements are described in the **Regulations of the Animal Welfare Act**.[33]

- Registration with USDA and adherence to USDA regulations is required by all institutions, except elementary or secondary schools, using cats in teaching, testing, or research in the United States.

- Unannounced, on-site inspection by veterinarians employed by the **Animal Care** section should be anticipated at least one a year and far more frequent visits are not uncommon.

- Requires an annual report of animal use covering the federal fiscal year from October 1 through September 31. The report is due by December 1.

The National Institutes of Health, Public Health Service (PHS)

- Oversight responsibility is described in the **Health Research Extension Act of 1985** (P.L. 99-158).[71]

- Policy is described in the Public Health Service Policy on Humane Care and Use of Laboratory Animals.[72] The Policy is administered through the Office for Protection from Research Risks (OPRR) with which an Assurance must be filed and approved.

- Adherence to the PHS Policy is required of those institutions conducting research using funds from PHS.

- Principles for implementation of PHS policy are those described in the *Guide for the Care and Use of Laboratory Animals.*[31]

The United States Food and Drug Administration (FDA) and the Environmental Protection Agency (EPA)

- Policies are described in the **Good Laboratory Practices for Nonclinical Laboratory Studies** (CFR 21 (Food and Drugs), Part 58, Subparts A-K; CFR Title 40 (Protection of Environment), Part 160, Subparts A-J; CFR Title 40 (Protection of Environment), Part 792, Subparts A-L).

- In general, standard operating procedures must be outlined and rigorously followed and supported with detailed records.

- Adherence is required when using cats in studies used to request research or marketing permits as part of the approval process for drugs or medical devices intended for human use.

Association for Assessment and Accreditation of Laboratory Animal Care International, Inc. (AAALAC International)

- AAALAC International is a nonprofit organization designed to provide peer review-based accreditation to animal research facilities.

- Basis for accreditation is adherence to principles described in the *Guide for the Care and Use of Laboratory Animals*.[31]

- Accreditation is voluntary with on-site inspections taking place every 3 years and annual reports being submitted.

In addition to the above regulatory bodies, state and local regulations may exist.

institutional animal care and use committee (iacuc)

The basic unit of an effective animal care and use program is the Institutional Animal Care and Use Committee (IACUC). The USDA, PHS, and AAALAC require an IACUC at any institution using cats in research, teaching, or testing. Important points regarding the composition of the IACUC include:

Number of members. USDA regulations require a minimum of three members, while the PHS policy requires a minimum of five members.

Qualifications of members. The IACUC should include the following:

- A chairperson

- A Doctor of Veterinary Medicine who has training or experience in laboratory animal medicine or science, and responsibility for activities involving animals at the research facility.

- An individual who is in no way affiliated with the institution other than as an IACUC member. At some institutions this role has been fulfilled by clergymen, lawyers, or local humane society or animal shelter officials.

In addition, PHS policy requires the following members:

- A practicing scientist with experience in animal research.

- One member whose primary concerns are in a non-scientific area. This individual may be an employee of the institution served by the IACUC.

It is acceptable for a single individual to fulfill more than one of the above categories.

Responsibilities of the IACUC. The written regulations should be consulted for an in-depth description of IACUC responsibilities. In general, the IACUC is charged with the following:

- Review of proposed protocols for activities involving use of animals in research, teaching, and testing. Protocols must be approved by the IACUC before animal use may begin.

- Semi-annually, inspect and assure that the animal research facilities and all animal care programs meet the standard of the regulations.

- Assure that personnel are adequately trained and qualified to conduct research using animals.

- Assure that animals are properly handled and cared for.

- Assure that the investigator has considered alternatives to potentially painful or stressful procedures and has determined that the research is nonduplicative.

- Assure that sedatives, analgesics, and anesthetics are used when appropriate.

- Assure that proper surgical preparation and technique are utilized.

- Assure that animals are euthanized appropriately.

cat quality

When cats are used in research, variables involving the cats will impact the scientific data collected from them. Ideally, the only experimental variables experienced by the animals during the project would be through the experimental manipulation. However, this ideal situation cannot be practically attained as all influences on the cats cannot be precisely controlled. For instance, there are differences between food batches, not all the animals are genetically and behaviorally identical, husbandry care will vary from day to day and person to person, noise and bacterial loads in the environment will change. One of the goals of the animal facility is to minimize variations in as many of these factors as is practical. When procuring animals for research, controlling variables within the animals must be considered.[73]

Note: Animal variability should be minimized to the extent practical considering the sensitivity of the intended research to the recognized animal variables.

Sources

There are two general sources of cats: **in-house bred** and **commercially purchased**.

1. **In-house breeding** of cats can permit a high level of quality control as many influences on the cats can be controlled by the facility for the lifetime of the animal. Genetic, dietary, and disease control can be managed for the intended research. Such control can even include germ-free technology.[74] However, in-house breeding is management, labor, and cost intensive. Producing experimental groups, often of defined age and sex, on schedule for a specific project requires a large and intensively managed breeding colony. Breeding is discussed briefly elsewhere in this volume, but breeding is not a simple activity. In-house breeding, while valuable for quality control, is rarely cost effective and is generally limited to very specialized research.

2.   **Commercial vendors** are generally the main source of
supply of cats for research. These vendors may produce
cats through breeding programs or acquire cats which
they then resell for research. The former are licensed by
the USDA as Class A Dealers. Cats thus bred for research
have a potential to be extremely high quality as many of
the influences on the animals can be controlled as with
in-house breeding programs. The cats have a known
medical and husbandry history. Their age and familial
associations are known. Depending on the vendor's colony management, they may have fairly high genetic and
temperamental uniformity. Age and sex-matched experimental groups are generally available (although it must
be remembered that cats have long reproductive cycles
and small litter sizes; and therefore, their availability is
much more restricted than for laboratory rodents).

> **Note:**   One of the primary considerations in cat colony man-
> agement and research use is feline infectious diseases.

Many feline infectious diseases are chronic infections
that may flare up under stress, affecting research being
conducted at the time. Vendors producing cats through
breeding colonies have the opportunity to eliminate these
diseases thereby making available animals free of a
potentially significant and uncontrolled experimental
variable. Colony control of feline herpesvirus has been
described.[75] Cats from colonies free of infectious diseases
are generally referred to as "specific pathogen-free" or
"SPF" cats. SPF cats are generally "barrier-housed."

Vendors that resell cats acquired from other sources are
licensed by the USDA as **Class B Dealers**. These vendors may
buy cats from breeders, other Class B dealers and from animal
pounds and shelters. Generally, the cats' medical and living
histories are unknown. Their ages are often general estimates.
The cats are often procured from a variety of sources and may
include cats from well-managed home-based breeders to feral
animals captured by animal control officials. Infectious diseases

are commonly carried by these cats and there is a high potential for cross-infection when they are gathered together in the dealer's facility. The dealers are required to hold the animals for a period prescribed by the Animal Welfare Act before they are sold to the research facility; however, the required time may vary depending on the animal's source and it is not based on disease management. Therefore, while these cats from random sources can make good research candidates, the potential for experimental variability from animal factors, and infectious diseases most notably, is quite high. Class B vendors often prepare the cats for the research environment making them better laboratory animals. This process is called "conditioning."

Note: "SPF", "barrier-housed", and "conditioned" labels are generic terms that can be defined differently by different vendors. Prior to acquiring cats from a vendor, a facility should inquire about the vendor colony management so that these terms can be interpreted.

Quarantine and Conditioning

All cats, regardless of source, should be quarantined and conditioned by the research facility prior to use. The exact procedures used must be designed with consideration for the initial quality of the vendor, the intended research use, and the facility's colony situation.

- SPF cats from reputable vendors may require only physical examination and a short holding period for stabilization to the new facility.

- Random source cats may require much more extensive quarantining and conditioning procedures.

- Cats brought into a facility without other cats may be handled differently than in a facility with pre-existing cat colonies.

- Cats intended for short, low-stress research projects may be handled differently than cats intended for survival surgical procedures.

The quarantining and conditioning process should be designed by the attending veterinarian, but it may include such things as:

- Examination of the shipping documents to assure that they are accurate and complete.

- Examination by technical staff to assess whether the cat meets the animal order specifications, such as correct sex (Figure 5). Obvious medical or behavioral problems should be noted.

- Physical examination by the attending veterinarian to help detect less obvious medical problems.

- Abdominal palpation or other procedures to assess pregnancy.

- Serology, bacterial culture, blood smear examination, fecal flotation and culture to assess past infectious disease exposure, and potential for disease carriage.[76-80]

- Vaccination for common feline diseases such as panleukopenia, pneumonitis, and rhinotracheitis.

- Treatment for common external and internal parasites.[81] Infection with a wide variety of parasites should be anticipated in random-source cats.[82]

- Housing period to allow the cats to physiologically stabilize to new diets, lighting cycles, human, and other environmental exposures. Each facility must develop its own guidelines based on it's cat use but 7 days is typical.

- Quarantining period, with isolation from pre-existing colony cats, to allow incubating diseases to manifest. Each facility must develop its own guidelines based on the factors discussed above and the period may range from as little as 0 days to as much as 60 days.

occupational health and zoonotic diseases

Animals present health risks that workers should be made aware.[83] Animal source is an important variable in the risks

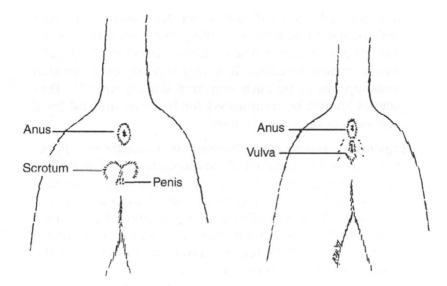

FIG. 5. Sex identification of the adult cat. Palpation for the penis is often helpful when verifying the sex.

involved; cats purchased from reputable animal breeders being of much lower risk for many zoonotic diseases than cats procured from random sources. The zoonotic diseases of cats have been reviewed elsewhere.[84] The need for and aspects of comprehensive programs for occupational health and medicine for individuals working with laboratory animals, have been described.[83,85-88] In general, personnel should be educated about the risks involved, wear a clean lab coat or coveralls when working with research animals and notify medical personnel of their potential exposures. Occupational health programs for personnel handling cats should be developed with consideration for the following occupational hazards.

Bite and scratch wounds. Research cats should be chosen partially on the basis of their behavior and cats with a propensity to bite and scratch should be avoided. Claw tips often can be clipped to help avoid injuries to handlers. Bites and scratches should be thoroughly washed as soon as practical. Cat bites frequently become infected, with *Pasteurella multocida* frequently isolated.[89] In addition to local infections of cat scratch wounds, a systemic infection called Cat Scratch Disease presents with regional lymphnode swelling and pain 1 to 2 weeks following a scratch.[90] The causative bacteria, *Bartonella (Rochalimaea) henselae*, has only recently been isolated and appears to be fairly common among cats.[91,92] Personnel should be immunized for tetanus, and rabies if random-source cats are used.

Ringworm. Ringworm is the common name for skin infections with fungi called dermatophytes. The dermatophyte, *Microsporum canis*, is most commonly associated with infections acquired from cats.[93] In humans and cats, lesions are typically circular, red, and crusty lesions that itch; however, cats frequently fail to show evidence for the disease.[93] Colony management to eliminate the disease has been proposed.[93,94]

Other skin lesions. Another fungus, *Sporothrix schenckii*, can be acquired from cats. While it is an uncommon disease, cats are frequently the source. It causes skin nodules and draining wounds in both cats and humans.[93] Mild but itchy skin lesions can also be secondary to infestations by the cat flea, *Ctenocephalides felis*, and the fur mite, *Cheyletiella blakei*.[95] These problems would not be anticipated from cats bred for research by quality vendors.

Toxoplasmosis. Cats are the definitive host of the intestinal protozoa, *Toxoplasma gondii*. The infection may be severe in kittens.[96] Following infection, oocysts are shed in the feces, usually for 1 to 2 weeks.[97,98] The oocysts must sporulate before they become infectious to humans. Human infections have been reviewed.[99] The primary concern being that human feti can be severely affected if pregnant women are exposed to *Toxoplasma*.[98,99] While infection in the research environment is unlikely, particularly with purpose-bred cats, many facilities avoid assigning pregnant women to cat care. Cats can be tested for serological evidence for past infection.[100]

Q Fever. Another protozoan infection acquired from cats is Q fever caused by *Coxiella burnetii*.[101,102] The disease is more commonly associated with contact with ruminants but infections have occurred following exposure to birth fluids of cats.[103] The infection is usually a flu-like syndrome but it may be severe and even fatal. Due to the extremely high infectiousness of the organism, people may be infected that are exposed via environmental contamination.

Intestinal zoonoses. Cat feces can contain bacteria that are infectious to humans. *Salmonella spp.* and *Campylobacter* may both infect cats and be shed in the feces. One study found over half of cats to be culture positive for *Campylobacter.*[104] The isolates from cats have been typed as the same bacteria as those found in human enteritis.[105] Campylobacteria may also cause diarrhea in the infected cats.[106] The intestinal protozoa, *Giardia,* is also found but the zoonotic nature of the cat isolate has been questioned.[107,108]

Dysgonic fermenter-type 2. Dysgonic Fermenter-type 2 (DF-2) is speciated as *Capnocytophaga canimorsus.* It is a gram-negative bacillus that is part of the normal oral flora of dogs and cats, is responsible for increasing numbers of cases of fulminant septicemia in humans.[109] Patients usually have preexisting medical illnesses, but infection also occurs in otherwise healthy individuals. Infection is generally from a bite wound. It does not cause clinical signs in dogs or cats. In humans, it causes local infection (cellulitis), septicemia, meningitis, polyarthritis, osteomyelitis, and bacterial endocarditis. Most systemic human cases have been in immunosuppressed or splenectomized individuals and mortality is high.

Rabies. This viral encephalitis is lethal in both humans and cats. There is virtually no risk of rabies from purpose-bred research cats but random source animals could be infected prior to acquisition, even with fairly long conditioning periods.[110] Vaccination of personnel exposed to random source cats is recommended.

Allergy. Allergies to cats are not uncommon in personnel exposed to cats. The primary allergen from cats has been found to be a salivary protein, Fel d 1.[111] Personnel may experience respiratory symptoms such as sneezing and rhinitis or skin symptoms such as redness, swelling, and pruritis following exposure. As with many other allergies, the symptoms can interfere with the person's ability to function in their chosen job and thus represents a serious occupational hazard. It is advisable for personnel to wear a face mask or fitted respirator, gloves, and a clean, launderable lab coat or coveralls. In addition, it is advisable for animal care workers to undergo periodic respiratory function testing. Ideally, sensitive personnel should be reassigned to job tasks which eliminate the possibility of exposure to allergens. Reassignment to areas away from cats maybe helpful but cat allergy is a risk factor for rat and mouse allergy, as well.[112]

Experimental biohazards. The research studies conducted on the cats may introduce chemical, radioactive and infectious hazards into the workplace. In such cases, it is recommended that standard operating procedures for safe handling of biohazardous materials and contaminated animals be established and followed. Guidelines for use of biohazardous agents are discussed in detail elsewhere.[83]

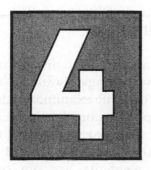

veterinary care

basic veterinary supplies

The following basic supplies are useful for the clinical care of cats:

1. A stethoscope.

2. Disposable syringes, ranging in size from 1 mL to 12 mL.

3. Disposable hypodermic needles, ranging in size from 21 to 26 gauge (diameter)and 5/8 to 1 1/2 inch (length).

4. Blood collection tubes with no additive (for serum) or added EDTA (for wholeblood).

5. Gauze sponges.

6. Small-animal rectal thermometer.

7. Lubricating jelly.

8. Disinfectant such as povidone-iodine solution.

9. Sterile fluids such as lactated Ringer's solution or 0.9% sodium chloride.

10. Nail clippers.

11. Bacterial culture swabs in transport media.

12. Additional supplies should supplement those listed above depending upon theneeds of the facility.

physical examination

Cats should be examined upon arrival in the research facility and a record of those findings should be included in the cat's medical record. This baseline examination is useful to determine if the cat meets the specifications for the facility and the research project, as well as for comparison should the cat become ill at a later date. Physical examination should always be done systematically so that elements are not overlooked. A useful sequence of examination is as follows:

- The feces and urine in the cage pan should be inspected, and abnormal consistency, color, or odor noted.

- The feed and water bowls should be checked to evaluate the cat's appetite.

- General assessment of behavior of the animal within the cage and during removal from the cage. Findings such as lethargy or aggressiveness should be noted.

- The eyes should be examined for discharge or abnormal reddening of the conjunctiva.

- The nose should be examined for discharge.

- The lips and mouth should be examined for lesions and mucous membrane color.

- The ears should be examined for accumulation of dry, brown, crusty material, which is suggestive of ear mite infestation.

- The coat should be examined for hair loss and skin lesions.

- The body should be felt for subcutaneous masses, lymphnode enlargements, and skeletal abnormalities.

- The perineal region is examined for fecal or urine staining, sex determination, vulvar discharge, and for open or closed lesions.

- A stethoscope should be used to listen for abnormal respiratory sounds and for the heart rate and sounds.

- The abdomen should be palpated for masses. This is particularly important for assessing pregnancy in random-source cats. Palpation is performed by standing directly behind the cat and firmly pressing the fingers of both hands into the cranial part of the abdomen and slowly drawing the fingers back caudally or by standing to the side of the cat and grasping the abdomen from the ventral surface while letting the viscera slip upward away from your fingers (Figure 6).

- The body temperature should be measured. This should be done last as cats frequently rebel against the procedure. Two techniques can be used. The most common method involves a small-animal glass rectal thermometer, which has had a small amount of lubricating jelly applied to the bulb, inserted 2 to 4 cm into the rectum. Alternatively, the body temperature may be measured from the ear by use of an infrared tympanic thermometer.[113] While the technique is very fast and is well accepted by cats, several trials should be performed per cat as repeatability can be a problem.

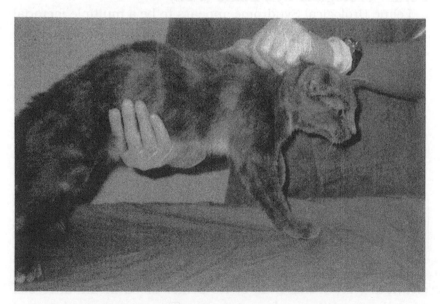

FIG. 6. Abdominal palpation of the cat.

common clinical problems

This section briefly describes common clinical problems of research colony cats. Many clinical problems appear similar initially and there are frequently extenuating circumstances that must be considered when therapy is developed. Two concerns that must be considered with research cats are maintaining a high level of health in the animal group and understanding how the research activities are related to the health problem. These concerns often transcend the importance of the individual ill cat's problem. Treating ill cats is required for humane, legal, and experimental reasons; however, all illnesses should be viewed as evidence of potential management failures. Diseases have overt physiological effects that can influence or nullify research results and are often avoidable in the controlled research setting. Laboratory animal veterinarians have specialized training in colony management and research influences, and thus, veterinary expertise should be sought whenever clinical problems develop.

Feline Urological Syndrome (FUS)

Feline Urological Syndrome appears to be a multiple factorial problem of the urinary tract of cats.[114] A common subset of this syndrome is urolithiasis. Urolithiasis refers to the development of mineral concretions within the urinary tract. This leads to urinary bladder inflammation, blood in the urine, and frequent attempts to urinate. The concretions are composed of sand-like material containing magnesium ammonium phosphate and proteinaceous material and are called struvite uroliths.[46] Particularly in male cats, this material can lodge in the urethra causing an obstruction to the passage of urine.

Note: Urethral obstruction is a medical emergency and veterinary attention must be obtained at once.

Cats with urethral obstruction will make frequent attempts of urinate, producing little or no urine. Blood in the litter box or at the tip of the penis is common. The cats are restless and may vocalize from discomfort.

Clinical disease problems with urolithiasis can be minimized through good colony management. Since the minerals from which the crystals are formed originate in the diet, food and water management are key tools for minimizing urinary tract problems. Much research has been done on the relationship between diet and urolithiasis so high-quality diets from reputable food vendors will be formulated with this knowledge base.

- **Minerals.** In general, while the mineral components of struvite originate in the diet, the total mineral content of the diet is not particularly important.[45] Older literature commonly implicates magnesium levels in the diet; however, it has been found that the acceptable magnesium level in diets is very broad.[37]

- **pH.** The pH of the urine is influenced by the diet components, with plant products tending to induce alkaline urine, and pH is a critical factor in the formation of struvite.[45] When urine pH is maintained below 6.4, struvite will rarely form.[45]

- **Urine concentration.** The other important factor in struvite formation is urine concentration. Urine can contain struvite minerals at levels of approximately twice their solubility without precipitation[45] so maintenance of good hydration of the cats is important. Some cats are reticent to drinking water and other techniques may need to be employed for supply them with greater fluid intake. It has been found that total fluid intake is greater in cats fed canned diets than in cats fed dry chow.[38,46]

- **Prevention.** Cats with a history of urolithiasis should be put on a high quality, meat-based, canned cat food.

Retroviral Diseases

There are two notable retroviral diseases of cats: **Feline Leukemia Virus** (FeLV) and **Feline Immunodeficiency Virus** (FIV). A recent survey of random source cats found infection rates at about 5%.[115]

FIV has been reviewed in more detail elsewhere.[116] It is a lentivirus first identified in 1986. In experimental infection, kittens demonstrate transient fever 1 to 2 months after infection and lymphadenopathy for up to 9 months. Most infected cats become lifelong carriers and some cats develop a terminal AIDS-like syndrome. The infection is most prevalent in free-roaming cats, the common origin of random source cats. Transmission appears to be through bites as intimate, non-traumatic contact in laboratory settings has failed to demonstrate transmission.[116-118]

FeLV was first isolated in 1964. It is a C-type RNA virus and causes lymphosarcoma in some infected cats. Following infection, some cats develop immunity while others become persistently infected. In addition to lymphosarcoma, the infection is associated with other neoplasms, immunodeficiency disorders, bone marrow suppression, glomerulonephritis, and reproductive abnormalities.

These retroviral infections, particularly FeLV, are contributory to clinical disease from a wide variety of other diseases.[119-121] Subtle physiologic effects of these infections should be expected in the absence of clinical disease.[122-124] The impact of these chronic infections on superimposed research is impossible to predict but some effects should be anticipated. Tests and testing recommendations have recently been reviewed.[125,126]

Abscesses

Cats that have physical contact with other cats periodically fight. These fights may appear quite minor, but quick bites and scratches may deposit bacteria below the skin surface. These can develop into abscesses in the ensuing days and weeks. Abscesses appear as fluctuant swellings that may be warm or draining. Inappetance and fever are commonly seen. Mixed bacterial infections are common as is *Pasteurella multocida*. While antibiotic therapy can be a useful adjuvant, the primary treatment is by establishing drainage.

Dermatophytosis (Ringworm)

Ringworm is a dermal infection with a fungus; most commonly this is caused by *Microsporum canis* in cats.[93] Infection may be subclinical or characterized by hair loss, reddening of the skin, and crusts or scabs on the face, ears, and forelimbs. The lesions sometimes itch and the cats may scratch at them. Diagnosis is made by clinical appearance, culture of hairs at the lesion margins on dermatophyte test media (DTM), or by

microscopic examination of lesion skin scrapings mounted in
10% KOH for typical dermatophyte organisms. The organism
will infect humans, as well. Treatment should entail systemic
administration of griseofulvin or itraconazole.[127] Topical treatments may not be effective.[128]

Ear Mites

The cat ear mite, *Otodectes cynotis*, causes irritation to the
ear canal. Infested cats scratch their ears and have excessive,
black exudate in the ear. With careful observation, white specks
may be seen moving over the surface of the exudate. A definitive
diagnosis of the mite may be made by smearing the exudate on
a slide and observing under low-power microscopy for the mite.
Daily cleaning with mineral oil for 10 to 14 days or a single
treatment with 400 microgram Ivermectin/kg body weight SQ
are usually effective in eliminating the organism. Colony-wide
treatment and sanitation should be explored to reduce the possibility of re-occurrence.

Intestinal Parasitism

A variety of intestinal parasites infest cats. Intestinal parasitism is primarily a problem of random-source cats. Clinical disease is not often seen in adult cats but more severe problems
can develop in intensive rearing environments. The parasites
can also complicate research, especially involving the gastrointestinal tract. Identification of the worms by fecal ova examination is recommended so that the appropriate drugs can be
used for treatment.

Fleas

The cat flea, *Ctenocephalides felis*, is often hard to detect on
cats due to their fastidious grooming. Flea infestations are a
problem of random-source cats. Treatment usually entails dip-
ping or dusting with pyrethrum-based insecticides. Treatment
must be carefully chosen to avoid toxicity to the cat and with
consideration of the potential research effects of the chemicals
used.

Respiratory Infections

A wide variety of respiratory diseases infect cats. These are a
common and persistent problem whenever cats are intensively

housed. Mycoplasma may be important lower respiratory pathogens in cats.[129] Feline Herpes Virus, Feline Calicivirus, *Bordetella bronchiseptica*, and Chlamydia are the more commonly recognized upper respiratory pathogens. Surveys have found that the disease prevalence rates can exceed 80%.[130] Elimination of these diseases should be a primary focus of specific pathogen-free feline vendors as infected cats may become persistent carriers of the organisms.[131] As carriers, they may shed the organisms to other cats and they may develop clinical disease when stressed. Infections often present as epidemics with several animals ill at one time and with the infections sweeping from animal to animal. Disease will manifest as conjunctivitis, sneezing, ocular and nasal discharges, fever, and anorexia. For research purposes, it is important to recognize that these diseases have broad physiological effects that may interfere with many kinds of studies.[132] Vaccination is helpful in reducing the seriousness of the infections when administered before an outbreak. Depending on the organism involved and the presence of secondary infections, antibiotic therapy can be helpful in treatment but often supportive nursing care is most needed.[133] The management aspects of respiratory diseases have been reviewed.[29]

Feline Infectious Peritonitis (FIP)

FIP has been a persistent problem in intensively raised cats. It is caused by a coronavirus that chronically infects. The virus is shed most commonly through feces and oropharyngeal secretions, especially early in the course of infection. The consequences of infection are quite variable, from not detectable to chronic debilitation and lethal peritonitis, making diagnosis difficult. The disease has been reviewed.[134,135] There are two major forms of FIP. An **effusive form** characterized by high protein fluid accumulation in body cavities and a **noneffusive form** characterized by pyogranulomatous lesions in any body organ or system. Signs common to both forms of FIP include fluctuating antibiotic-unresponsive fever, lethargy, anorexia, and weight loss. Stress, crowding, poor sanitation, parasitism, and concurrent diseases, particularly immunosuppressive diseases such as feline leukemia virus (FeLV) and feline immunodeficiency virus (FIV), may increase the impact of FIP virus on cats. In laboratory colonies, the disease must be distinguished from the closely related enteric corona viruses which cause transient infections.[136] From a research perspective, the disease would be anticipated to broadly effect infected animals rendering the experimental results suspect.[137,138]

Enteric Diseases (Diarrhea)

Enteric diseases are common problem of cats, especially random source cats. Clinical signs of disease are not typically seen; however, problems may develop in intensive housing situations and when the animals are stressed by experimentation. Intestinal infections generally manifest as diarrhea if outward signs are seen. A number of infectious agents can infect the intestinal tract of cats. Rotavirus, Feline Enteric Coronavirus, and parasites such as coccidia, tapeworms, and round worm will infect and may cause clinical disease. Other organisms will infect cats and may spread to humans as well, these include *Giardia* species, *Salmonella* species, and *Campylobacter jejuni*.[104] The most overtly pathogenic agent is Feline Panleukopenia Virus. This parvovirus causes serious disease, commonly causes death, and is often called "feline distemper". It is persistent in the environment and colonies must be managed to control this disease. Vaccination is effective when used in accordance with appropriate colony management.

Metabolic Disorders

An unusual metabolic disorder of hepatic metabolism of protein and lipid has been seen in cats, including research cats.[139] The cause has not yet been determined but nutritional support appears to be the best therapy available. The disease has been reviewed.[140] Cats seem to have an unusual propensity to develop hyperthyroidism. This is condition of older cats (>9 years) manifesting as weight loss with an increased appetite. Affected cats often have an ill-kempt appearance. A similar presentation is seen in cats that develop diabetes mellitus. Increased drinking and urination is also characteristic. Each of these metabolic disorders require complex veterinary medical management that is difficult to balance with the research use.

Implant Problems

Cats are frequently used in research entailing implantation of catheters or electrodes. The research devices are associated with a variety of medical problems. Great care must be taken in planning projects involving long-term implants in an effort to minimize these problems. The most common problems are associated with infection. The procedures for use of these devices must include scrupulous adherence to sterile technique during placement, efficacious sterilization of the devices prior to implantation, careful exit-site and implant nursing care to assure minimal contamination and judicious use of antibiotics.[17] Implants that become infected frequently fail to function and generally become a nidus of infection if antibiotic treatments are discontinued.

Note: It is often the best course of management to remove the implant once it becomes infected.

---

treatment of disease

Treatment of sick cats should be implemented under the direction of a qualified veterinarian, following appropriate diagnostic measures. A short list of drugs which can be used in cats is provided in Table 7. Abbreviations for route of administration are PO (oral), IV (intravenous), IM (intramuscular), and SC (subcutaneous). Abbreviations for frequency of administration are SID (once daily), and BID (twice daily).

General Treatment of Dehydration

Cats frequently become dehydrated. Most cats drink little water routinely and ill cats consume even less. Some conditions, such as diarrhea, increase fluid loss and dehydration can rapidly become severe. Treatment should replace lost fluid and electrolytes, regardless of the precise etiology. The severity of dehydration can be assessed by the "skin-tent" test, in which a fold of skin on the dorsum of the neck is lifted and released. Ordinarily, the lifted skin should return within 1 second; however, if the

TABLE 7. DRUGS DOSAGES FOR CATS

Drug	Dosage information	General application	Reference
Dexamethasone	0.125–0.5 mg/kg, IM	Shock, anti-inflammatory	141
Prednisolone	2–4 mg/kg, PO every other day	Anti-inflammatory	141
Doxapram	5–10 mg/kg IV	Stimulation of respiratory activity	141
Piperazine	1.9 g/kg PO, repeat in 10–21 days	Endoparasites	141
Mebendazole	22 mg/kg SID for 3 days	Endoparasites	142
Oxytocin	5–10 units IM or SC	Stimulation of uterine contractions	141
Kaolin-pectin suspension	1–2 mL/kg PO every 2–6 hours	Diarrhea	143
Griseofulvin	65 mg/kg PO SID 6 weeks	Dermatophytosis	141
Amoxicillin	11–22 mg/kg PO BID	Bacterial infections	143
Cephalexin	35 mg/kg PO BID	Bacterial infections	141
Tetracycline	25 mg/kg PO BID	Bacterial infections	17
Procaine penicillin G	40,000 IU/kg IM SID	Bacterial infections	143
Enrofloxacin	5 mg/kg IM SID	Bacterial infections	144
Gentamicin	4.4 mg/kg SC or IM SID	Bacterial infections	143

animal is dehydrated, it will fall into place more slowly. In severe cases, the "tent" may stand over 10 seconds.

In general, appropriate replacement fluids should be isotonic. Saline at 0.9%, 5% dextrose, and lactated Ringers Solution are commonly administered fluids. It is important to assess hydration of the animal while it is receiving fluids, since over-administration of fluids can lead to serious complications. As a general guideline, fluids may be given in increments of 30 to 40 mL/kg of body weight until normal hydration is achieved. Fluids are most easily administered subcutaneously. Intravenous administration is also practical.

General Treatment of Anorexia

Cats may experience anorexia for a number of reasons, however the specific cause is not always discernible. Although any specific cause should be appropriately eliminated following diagnostic identification, it is also appropriate to engage nonspecific measures to encourage cats to eat and thereby overcome anorexia. An important aspect of eating for cats is food odor. Cats experiencing respiratory disease with nasal discharges will sometimes eat if their nose is kept clean. Cats can also be enticed to begin eating by offering a variety of foods. Meat flavored, specialty canned diets can be tried, as well as warming the food. Commercially available nutritional supplements (e.g., Nutrical®, Evsco Pharmaceuticals, Buena, NJ) can be administered orally. Treatment for anorexia and nutritional management of ill cats has been reviewed elsewhere.[145,146] Animals which experience significant loss of body condition in the face of prolonged, unresolving anorexia should be humanely euthanized.

General Treatment of Open Skin Lesions

Cats may develop open skin lesions for a variety of reasons, including trauma and abscesses related to bacterial infection. In all cases, it is important to keep the lesion free of contaminating debris. In addition, it is advisable to clean all open lesions at least once a day with an antiseptic solution such as betadine.

Whether or not the inciting cause of the lesion was a bacterial pathogen, any open wound is susceptible to secondary bacterial infection. For this reason, application of a topical bacterial ointment should be considered. In addition, it is advisable to perform bacterial culture on lesions which demonstrate drainage suggestive of infection. Systemic antibiotic therapy should be based on the outcome of culture and antibiotic sensitivity testing.

It is unwise to attempt to suture or otherwise close draining lesions. To the contrary, drainage should be permitted as part of the normal healing process.

Disease Prevention Through Sanitation

Practicing proper sanitation is the best way to control many diseases of the cat. Cat cages should be routinely cleaned and disinfected as described in Chapter 2. Efforts should be made to prevent excessive accumulation of feces, urine and dander both in the cage and in the room. Instruments and equipment used on more than a single animal should be cleaned and disinfected between cats. In addition, use of disposable gloves will facilitate control of infectious disease. Personnel should wash their hands with an antiseptic soap after handling cats suspected of harboring infectious agents. Optimally, cats infected with pathogens should be isolated from noninfected animals.

anesthesia and analgesia

One of the foremost concerns in animal research is protecting the subjects from unnecessary pain and distress. It is critically important that anesthesia and analgesia be provided with all the care and expertise possible. These critical subjects are reviewed briefly here but detailed information is readily available and should be sought by investigators involved in potentially painful or distressful procedures.

Proper use of pain alleviating drugs involves sophisticated control of all key physiological systems (nervous, cardiovascular, and respiratory systems). General anesthesia profoundly affects the physiological state of the anesthetized animal. A plethora of factors influence the process each time it is performed. Health of the animal can have a major impact. An animal that appears quite normal on initial inspection may have conditions that can lead to uncontrolled anesthesia and death. A procedure area that is cold can dramatically change the manner that an animal will react to administered drugs. An individual animal's response to an anesthetic drug will vary during a procedure in response to the research manipulations as well as it's changing physiological state. It is known that age, sex, strain, previous drug exposure, and even time of day of exposure can have important impacts on anesthetic drug responses. The knowledge of physiology and pharmacology required for precisely managed anesthesia is enormous. This required expertise is recognized in clinical medicine by highly trained and specifically certified physicians and veterinarians. Conversely, in the research environment, persons administering anesthetics may have only cursory training in these areas. Fortunately through the use of modern drugs with wide safety margins and the impressive resilience of healthy animals, anesthesia in the research setting is generally quite routine. However, always remember that anesthesia is a complex system and many factors can abruptly crop up to cause serious problems. Training by and frequent consultation with the attending veterinarian is advisable.

Definitions Commonly Used in Animal Anesthesia

Analgesia.   Loss of sensation of pain.

Anesthesia.   Total loss of sensation in a part or in the whole body, generally induced by the administration of a drug that depresses nervous tissue activity.

Local anesthesia.   Loss of sensation limited to a local area.

General anesthesia.   Loss of consciousness and loss of sensation throughout the body.

Surgical anesthesia.   Loss of consciousness and sensation with sufficient muscle relaxation and analgesia to allow surgery to be performed without pain or struggling.

Dissociative anesthesia.   A central nervous system state characterized by muscular rigidity, peripheral analgesia and altered consciousness (e.g., ketamine anesthesia).

Balanced anesthesia.   Surgical anesthesia produced by a combination of two or more drugs or anesthetic techniques each contributing differing pharmacological effects.

Terminal surgery. The animal is anesthetized, a procedure is performed and euthanasia is conducted before the animal regains consciousness.

Survival surgery. Procedure performed with the intent of recovering the animal to consciousness from the anesthesia.

Major surgery. Procedures involving exposure of a body cavity or which creates a permanent physical or physiological impairment.

Minor surgery. Surgical procedures that do not meet the definition of Major.

Controlled substances. Drugs regulated by the Drug Enforcement Administration; classified according to abuse potential.

Neuroleptanalgesia. Hypnosis and analgesia produced by a combination of a neuroleptic drug and an analgesic drug.

Sedation. A mild degree of central nervous system depression in which the patient is awake but calm. The patient may be aroused with sufficient stimuli. Sedatives act by dose dependent depression of the cerebral cortex.

Tranquilization. A state of tranquillity and calmness in which the patient is relaxed, awake and unconcerned with its surroundings. With sufficient stimuli the patient is aroused. Analgesia is not a component of tranquilization. Tranquilizers act by depressing the hypothalamus and the reticular activating system.

Choosing an Anesthesia Regimen

When choosing anesthetic agents consideration must be given to providing appropriate depth and length of anesthesia and analgesia as determined by the procedure. The agents used should be safe and effective for the species under study given its age, sex, history, and physical condition. The agent should also be safe and relatively convenient for the personnel who are administering and monitoring anesthesia. Neuromuscular blocking agents are rarely necessary for surgery but they are sometimes necessary for specific research studies. These drugs are not anesthetics and they provide no analgesia. They paralyze animals making reflex monitoring for adequacy of anesthesia impossible. Therefore, neuromuscular blocking must be used only when necessary and they should be used only after experience has shown that the anesthetic regime is effective in the **absence** of the blocking agents.[147] Monitoring changes in blood pressure can be a helpful method of assessing anesthesia when these agents are used.

When choosing an anesthesia regimen careful consideration must be given to:

• The type of procedure being performed

• The duration of the procedure

• The amount and type of pain that may accompany the procedure

• The goals of the project

• The properties of the anesthetic

• The condition of the animal

Each agent has a different duration of action, length of recovery time, amount and site of analgesia, degree of muscle relaxation, site and route of detoxification or excretion, etc. The type of procedure also greatly influences the anesthesia requirements. Some procedures cause more pain than others. An understanding of the agents being used is also necessary to assure that they are safe for the species under study and that they will not interfere with the goals of the project. Drugs may be used in terminal procedures that are not appropriate for survival procedures.

The animal under study will also influence the anesthesia agents and route of administration. Tracheal intubation with inhalation anesthesia is the route of choice for most procedures. Tracheal intubation is quite easily mastered in cats.

It seems obvious that the health and general condition of the animal will affect the outcome of anesthesia but the investigator must be aware that animals may hide or compensate for disease processes to such an extent as to appear normal.

Understanding the anesthetic agent or agents that are to be used is extremely important in assuring success. Often an investigator's experience with a particular agent and the agent's previous use on a research project are the factors that determine its choice. Experience with an agent or anesthesia regime is important but it should not preclude consideration of other factors and consideration of new anesthesia regimes.

Pre-Anesthesia Evaluation

Prior to induction of anesthesia, animals should be carefully evaluated for good health.[148] If there are any doubts about the animal's health, anesthesia should not be initiated until a thorough veterinary exam has been conducted.

Care Prior to Anesthesia

The pre-anesthesia exam should be noted on an anesthesia record. Only healthy animals should be subjected to anesthesia for elective procedures. The following steps should be taken to assure that the animal is healthy prior to anesthesia:

- Confirmation of animal's number or other identification, sex, and age.

- Evaluation of a blood sample for hematological abnormalities.

- A brief physical examination including rectal temperature measurement and auscultation of the heart and lungs should be performed to assess the overall health status and to detect any signs of illness, particularly of respiratory disease.

- The animal should be weighed so that the accurate dose of anesthetic may be determined.

- Food and water should be removed at least 6 hours prior to induction of anesthesia. Withholding food from an animal (fasting) prior to induction of anesthesia is recommended with cats to reduce the incidence of vomiting and the potential for aspiration during anesthesia. It is not recommended to remove water sooner than this because it may lead to dehydration.

• For long and invasive procedures, an intravascular catheter should be secured for emergency drug delivery and for routine fluid administration. Sterile lactated Ringer's solution or 0.9% NaCl are appropriate fluids and should be administered at a dosage of 10 to 15 mL/kg of body weight per hour of anesthesia.

• To minimize production of respiratory secretions, which may interfere with respiration, glycopyrrolate (11 µg/kg IM) or atropine (0.05 mg/kg SC or IM) may be administered prior to anesthesia.[149]

• Assessment of body condition and general health. The body condition of the animal is very important to anesthesia induction, maintenance and recovery. Very thin animals may react rapidly to some agents and become overdosed at what should be an appropriate dosage. Very fat animals may be slow to respond to drugs.

• Estimate of hydration and assessment of mucous membrane color and capillary refill time. The skin and fur of an animal is a good indicator of the animal's general state of health. With practice, the skin can be used to roughly evaluate an animal's hydration status. If "pinched up" skin does not flatten out when released, the animal is dehydrated. Dry, tacky mucous membranes of the mouth are also an indication of dehydration. The color of the mucous membranes around the teeth should be pink. Mucous membranes, such as those lining the oral cavity, blanched by finger pressure should return to normal in 1 to 2 seconds.

• Gastrointestinal problems frequently cause changes to the stools. Stools should be noted as an assessment of the animal's health. Body temperature can be very useful as well.

TABLE 8.   EXAMPLE PRE-ANESTHETIC REGIMES

Drug	Dosage
Acepromazine	0.1–0.6 mg/kg SC or IM
Diazepam	0.2–0.4 mg/kg SC [a]
Midazolam	0.2–0.4 mg/kg SC or IM
Xylazine	0.4–1.1 mg/kg SC
Morphine	0.1 mg/kg SC or IM

[a] Repeated administration of diazepam has been associated with liver disease in cats.[150]

Pre-Anesthetic Medications

It is often advisable and sometimes necessary to premedicate an animal before induction of anesthesia. In general anticholinergic drugs, tranquilizers, and narcotics are used for premedication. Anticholinergic drugs are used to decrease oral and respiratory secretions; maintain the heart rate; and decrease gut motility. Tranquilizers relieve anxiety and produce calmness, aid in restraint, calm postoperative recovery, and reduce dose of anesthetic needed. Narcotics are used as preoperative medications to: quiet an animal; produce vomiting and defecation; reduce the amount of anesthesia needed; smooth recovery; and to provide postoperative pain relief. Following anesthetic induction, an ointment formulated for eye use should be used in the eyes to prevent them from drying out.

A variety of preanesthetic regimes are available for cats.[141,149] A short list of drugs which can be used in cats is provided in Table 8. Abbreviations for route of administration are IM (intramuscular) and SC (subcutaneous).

Administering Anesthesia

Injectable anesthesia   Certain agents can be given by the intramuscular (IM) and subcutaneous (SC or SQ) routes. Generally, these routes result in a slower induction time compared to the intravenous (IV) route. IM and SQ are often used for sedation and tranquilizing prior to induction of surgical anesthesia (see technical descriptions in Chapter 5). **Intramuscular** (IM) injection is relatively simple in cats. IM injections can be administered in any large muscle mass; the usual site is the back of the hind leg. Generally the site of injection need not be disinfected. The largest gauge (smallest diameter) needle that allows easy injection of the solution but that resists bending should be used. **Subcutaneous** (SQ) injections are simple in most animals. SQ injection deposits the injected substance in the space below the skin. This site is appropriate for administration of fluids when IV administration is not available. Irritating or hypertonic solutions should not be given SQ. As with IM injections, the needle size will depend upon the animal, viscosity of the solution and the volume needed. **Intraperitoneal** (IP) injections in cats lead to unpredictable dose responses and is not consistent with good veterinary practices.

Inhalation Anesthesia Inhalation anesthesia refers to vaporous agents that are delivered via the lungs. They have advantages and disadvantages when compared to injectable anesthesia regimes. The disadvantages include:

- Necessity of an adequate scavenger system to prevent human exposure

- Expense of a calibrated vaporizer

- Need for trained and experienced personnel to run anesthesia equipment.

The major advantages of inhalation anesthesia are:

- Rapid induction

- Rapid changes in level of anesthesia

- Safety for the animal (with experienced operator)

- Good analgesic effects and fewer adverse physiologic affects (generally speaking)

Note: In general, for long procedures and major operative procedures, inhalation anesthesia is the method of choice for anesthetizing cats.

Inhalation anesthesia is reviewed in greater detail elsewhere.[148] The two most commonly used drugs are halothane and isoflurane. They are similar agents; however, isoflurane experiences negligible biotransformation while a significant amount of halothane is transformed by the liver. Isoflurane also has fewer cardiovascular effects and permits very rapid changes in anesthetic depth. Newer inhalation agents have been reviewed in cats.[151] Nitrous oxide has some utility in feline inhalation anesthesia when supplied at 40 to 70% of total gas; however, it has quite low potency in cats and must be used with other more efficacious anesthetic agents.

Anesthesia may be induced with an injectable agent such as ketamine and then maintained with inhalation agents. The best method of maintaining anesthesia using inhalation agents is with a gas anesthesia machine and a non-rebreathing circuit.[148] Such machines have calibrated delivery vaporizers that deliver precise quantities of the anesthesia agent in oxygen. Anesthesia may be administered via a tight-fitting mask or nose cone or preferably though an endotracheal tube. If intubated with an endotracheal tube, the animal's ventilation can be supported and personnel exposure can be more readily limited.

All inhalation agents affect humans and may cause drowsiness and headaches. While unproved, chronic low level exposure appears to be associated with adverse health effects in humans.[148] Specific scavenging systems that draw waste anesthesia out of the building or that capture the agents are necessary. Personnel exposure limits are legally set at <2 ppm as a time-weighted average.[148]

Monitoring Anesthesia

Monitoring to assure that the level of anesthesia is adequate for the procedure being conducted is a major component of proper care. Monitoring the anesthetized animal involves four body systems: (1) the central and peripheral nervous system; (2) the respiratory system; (3) the cardiovascular system; and (4) the musculoskeletal system.[148] Normal values of heart rate and respiratory rate should be obtained prior to anesthesia.

- Monitoring depression of the **central nervous system** in an anesthetized patient takes experience. Basic patient parameters that should be evaluated throughout the operative procedure include: heart rate (pulse rate), rhythm and pulse intensity; respiratory rate, depth and character; mucous membrane color, capillary refill time; body temperature; muscle tone; and reflexes.

- Monitoring the **body temperature** throughout the operative procedure is extremely important. Anesthesia causes reduced muscular activity and depressed central thermoregulatory control leading to lowered body temperature. Peripheral perfusion is also decreased. Poor circulation and hypothermia potentiate anesthesia and increase recovery times. Care must be taken to maintain an animal's body temperature in a normal range. Thermal water circulating pads should be used whenever possible. Anesthetized animals should always be placed on towels or pads, never directly on stainless steel tables. Animals should never be placed directly on a standard human heating pad. These pads can produce thermal burns even at low settings.

- **Heart rate** will generally decrease as the animal goes deeper under anesthesia and increase as they emerge from anesthesia. Rates below 100 beats per minute are cause for concern.[148]

- As with the heart rate, **respiratory rate** generally decreases (fewer breaths per minute) with depth of anesthesia. The breaths will initially become deep and regular in interval; they then become shallow and irregular. If the animal is getting "light" (i.e., moving towards awakening), respiration rate may increase and the breaths may appear shallow. In addition, a very light animal that is perceiving pain may consciously hold its breath.

- **Muscle tone** is an indicator of depth of anesthesia for agents other than ketamine (by itself).

- A variety of **reflexes** can be evaluated to monitor the depth of anesthesia.

  1. Reflexes of the eye are most commonly used. The eyelids will close (blink) when the cornea or eyelids are touched. These are the corneal and palpebral

reflexes, respectively. Generally, a brisk palpebral reflex is "too light" and a slow corneal is "too deep".

2. Withdrawal of the feet when stimulated shows the pedal or withdrawal reflex. Pinching the base of the toenail or the web of skin between the toes is the method used. If a toe pinch results in an increased heart rate, increased respiratory rate, movement of the animal's body or vocalization, the animal actually perceives the stimulation as pain and clearly, the anesthesia is insufficient.

*   **Pulse oximetry** can be a very useful method of monitoring as oxygen delivery and pulse rate can be conveniently and non-invasively measured.[152]

Note: Since different conditions can lead to similar presentations, it is imperative to track a variety of parameters throughout an operative procedure so that the trends can be used to evaluate each situation.

Anesthesia Recovery

The anesthesia recovery period commences at the end of the surgery and ends when the animal is fully awakened. In general, an unconscious animal should not be left unattended. When the animal reaches a semi-conscious state it should be monitored at least every 15 minutes.

Some drug effects can be reversed to speed recovery or to minimize adverse side effects.

*   **Doxapram** (0.2 mg/kg IV) increases respiratory effort and improves the state of arousal without antagonizing drugs specifically.

*   **Naloxone** (0.1 mg/kg IV) specifically antagonizes opioid drug effects (including analgesic effects).

*   **Butorphanol** (0.2–0.4 mg/kg IV) antagonizes opioid effects such as central nervous depression but offers some analgesic effects.

*   **Yohimbine** (0.4 mg/kg IV) will partially reverse the sedative effects of alpha adrenergic agonists such as xylazine.

A major component of postoperative care is monitoring and alleviating postoperative pain. The expected extent of postoperative pain, how that pain will be assessed and drugs that will be used to alleviate pain must be considered by both the investigator and the IACUC. Assessment of pain in cats requires careful observation of the animals and comparison of the findings with normal. In general, **pain is indicated by:**

- "Guarding" (protecting) the surgical site

- Vocalization (whining, growling, meowing) when the animal moves or if the surgical area is touched

- Limping, a "tucked-up" abdomen, or other abnormal stances or posture

- Reclusive behavior

- Lack of appetite

- Increased inspiratory rate or abnormal breathing patterns

Anesthesia Records

To assure that all aspects of anesthesia and surgery are conducted in an appropriate manner, written records must be maintained. The USDA regularly asks for anesthesia and postoperative care records. Even if the investigator keeps a logbook of animal procedures, complete records of preoperative evaluation and care, surgical monitoring, anesthesia recovery and post operative care must be maintained in the animal facility.

Suggested Anesthesia Regimes

There are a tremendous variety of anesthetic regimes for cats.[141,148,153-155] These typically involve general anesthesia by injection or inhalation. Local anesthesia can be useful and techniques for long-term epidural catheters have been described.[156] A limited list of anesthetic regimes are below in Table 9. Abbreviations for route of administration are IV (intravenous) and IM (intramuscular).

Pentobarbital has historically been widely used for research anesthesia. It is virtually never used in clinical veterinary practice

TABLE 9. ANESTHETIC REGIMES FOR CATS

Drug	Dosage	Reference
Propofol	2–6 mg/kg IV and 0.2–0.6 mg/kg/minute IV for maintenance (should be given with an analgesic agent)[a,b]	148
Ketamine with Acepromazine	2–6 mg/kg IV 0.4 mg/kg IV	148
Ketamine with Xylazine	2–6 mg/kg IV 6 mg/kg IV	148
Halothane by precision vaporizer	2–4% for induction and 0.5–1.5% for maintenance	148
Isoflurane by precision vaporizer	2.5–4.5% for induction and 1–3% for maintenance	148
Tiletamine with Zolezepam	7.5 mg/kg IM 7.5 mg/kg IM	152
Thiamylal	12–18 mg/kg IV	152
Urethane with halothane	1–1.3 g/kg 0.5%	153
Alpha Chloralose	60 mg/kg IV[c]	152

[a] Other authors have found that higher doses are required.[154]

[b] Severe side effects have been seen in cats when given repeatedly on consecutive days.[157]

[c] Following induction with a shorter acting agent; for use in non-recover procedures.

as better, safer drugs are available. It is irritating to tissues and hence should be administered intravenously. Pentobarbital should be dosed based on lean body mass and given to effect but generally the dosage would be approximately 30 mg/kg IV. Pentobarbital is a poor analgesic.

Ketamine is widely used in anesthesia of cats. Unlike most anesthetic drugs, it is not a central nervous system depressant and hence is characterized by increased muscle tone, swallowing reflexes and increased salivation. It is used as a pre-anesthetic and an anesthetic agent. For anesthesia, it is generally given with tranquilizer or sedative drugs. It has pretty good peripheral analgesic properties but visceral analgesia is poor.[148]

Analgesia Dosages

Analgesia use should always be considered when painful procedures, such as surgery, are performed. Since cats cannot directly describe their discomfort, pain must be inferred by observing the actions of the cat. Evidence for discomfort may be detected as changes in movement or posture, attention by the animal to the surgery area, aggression, protecting the area, or other behavioral changes. Cortisol and systolic blood pressure increases have also been found to be subtle indictors of pain.[158] Until recently, analgesic drugs have been used when such evidence for discomfort has been seen. Recently, **"pre-emptive analgesia"**, where analgesic drugs are used before pain is evidenced, has been found to be more effective for controlling pain.[148] Unless it is known that analgesia use will affect the research results, it is better to use analgesia when it is "not needed" and thereby give the animals the benefit of the doubt about whether our pain assessment is accurate. Several good general references are available on analgesia and drugs for pain relief.[159-162]

A variety of analgesia options are available for cats.[141,148,163,164,165] Example regimes for analgesia are listed in Table 10. Abbreviations for route of administration are PO (oral), IM (intramuscular), IV (intravenous), and SC (subcutaneous).

Note: The frequency of administration for analgesia is generally fairly variable and must be balanced for the intended effect and the observed response.

---

aseptic surgery

All survival surgery in cats must involve aseptic techniques and preparation of the surgical site. Generally, this involves the following procedures and principles:

- Hair at surgical sites is shaved with an electric clipper.

- The skin is scrubbed thoroughly with an antiseptic such as betadine scrub.

- The surgical site is isolated with sterile surgical drapes.

TABLE 10.   SUGGESTED ANALGESICS FOR CATS[a]

Drug	Dosage
Aspirin	10 mg/kg PO every 48 hours
Butorphanol	0.2–0.8 mg/kg IM every 2–6 hours
Buprenorphine	0.005–0.1 mg/kg IM every 6–12 hours
Flunixin meglumine	1.0 mg/kg SC (PO may also be effective) every 24 hours
Ketoprofen	0.5–1.0 mg/kg PO every 24 hours
Medetomidine	0.005–0.01 mg/kg IM every 1–4 hours
Morphine	0.1 mg/kg epidural, duration >10 hours
Morphine	0.05–0.2 mg/kg IV or IM every 1–4 hours
Oxymorphone	0.02–0.1 mg/kg IM every 2–4 hours
Pentazocine	1.0–2.0 IV or IM every 2–4 hours
Phenylbutazone	10–15 mg/kg PO every 8–12 hours
Xylazine	0.01–0.2 mg/kg IM or SC every 1–3 hours

[a] Only analgesic drugs and dosages specifically reported for use in cats should be used as many drugs, such as acetominophen, are toxic at dosages used in other species.

- Sterile surgical instruments are used for all surgical procedures.

- Individuals performing surgery or directly assisting the surgeon wear sterile surgical gloves, gowns, caps, and face masks.

- Principles of aseptic surgery are described in greater detail elsewhere.[166-170]

Note: Non-survival surgical procedures (those that do not involve recovery from anesthesia) need not be aseptic.

Postsurgical Management

Following surgery, animals should be monitored frequently until the experiment has been completed. Particular attention should be paid to the following:

- Any change in behavior or appetite should be noted. Changes may indicate that the animal is in pain or experiencing other complications.

- The edges of the surgical incision should remain neatly apposed, following surgery. Surgical sites must be examined to assure that cats do not remove sutures. Equipment such as **Elizabethan collars** may be useful to restrict the ability of the cat to bite sutures; however, many cats do not accept them. Sutures are typically removed after 10 to 14 days. **Tissue glue** is a useful alternative to sutures in cats, since the lack of a suture often diminishes the interest of the animal in the incision site.

- Signs of infection at the surgical site, in the days and weeks after surgery. Signs of infection include:

  1. Discharge, especially if thick or colored.

  2. Abnormal warmth, redness, or swelling.

  3. Elevated body temperature.

  Any discharge should be cultured for bacteria and antibiotic therapy begun under the guidance of a qualified veterinarian.

euthanasia

Euthanasia of animals should be conducted in a humane and professional manner. The specific method chosen should produce a quick, painless death. Individuals euthanizing cats should be properly trained in the euthanasia technique to be used and animals should be euthanized out of the sensory range of other animals.

Note: Assurance of euthanasia is critically important in all cases.

Very deeply anesthetized animals may appear dead; yet, they may recover from the anesthesia at a later time. Death should always be confirmed by stethoscopic auscultation for absence of a heartbeat. A convenient method of assuring euthanasia is to create a bilateral pneumothorax by permitting air to enter the chest cavity. This is best accomplished by making a small incision through each side of the chest.

A complete summary of recommendations for euthanasia can be found in the 1993 Report of the American Veterinary Medical Association Panel on Euthanasia.[171]

- The primary method of euthanasia for cats is by intra-vascular injection of a **barbiturate** overdose. A dose that is at least 3 times an anesthetic dose will be effective. Drug preparations specifically formulated for dog and cat euthanasia are readily available from veterinary supply vendors. However, they, as with pentobarbital, are controlled drugs under the regulations of the federal Drug Enforcement Administration.

- **Ketamine** is not acceptable for euthanasia when used alone but can be humane when used in conjunction with sedatives and tranquilizers. However, it is not very efficient as it requires very high doses.

- Cats may also be euthanized by overdose with **inhalant anesthetics** but drug delivery to protect personnel must be assured.

- **Carbon dioxide** inhalation can be used to euthanize cats in emergency situations but only following anesthesia with other agents, such as ketamine/xylazine.

---

notes

5

experimental methodology

This chapter is not intended to outline specific experimental uses but rather it describes basic information that is a foundation for many specific techniques. Cats have many features that make them unlike most other animals used in research. An appreciation and understanding of these special facets makes working with cats more successful.

cats as research models

Cats have a number of physiological peculiarities that should be considered when their use in research is contemplated. The evolutionary developments associated with the carnivorous diet should be considered. Since prey items readily supply arachidonate, taurine, arginine, niacin, and vitamin A, nutritional requirements for these have developed. Cats are intolerant of high-carbohydrate diets.[36] They select against diets containing saccharin, cyclomate, and casein[38] and are not attracted to the taste of sucrose.[36] Unique breed differences have also been seen.[7] Research that does not directly involve these peculiarities may still be influenced by their underlying metabolic origins.

Cats have a number of unique responses to chemicals making them different than other mammals. In general terms, cats have **slow hepatic biotransformation pathways**, they have **red blood cells that are unusually sensitive** to oxidation damage, and they have an unusual **sensitivity at certain drug receptor sites**. The metabolic pathways in the liver for glucuronide conjugation are defective. Cats are therefore quite sensitive to intoxication by aspirin, acetaminophen, phenolic compounds, alcohols, and aromatic carboxylic acids.[172] Common preservatives such as benzoate can cause problems.[37] The red blood cells of cats are unusually sensitive to oxidation damage. This seems to be due to a high sulfhydryl content and low methemoglobin reductase activity that normally repairs oxidative damage.[172] Propylene glycol, a common drug carrier and food additive, causes RBC oxidation and Heinz body anemia in cats.[173] Alloxan for chemical induction of diabetes mellitus is toxic in cats.[174] Repeated administration of diazepam and propofol have demonstrated toxic reactions.[150,157] Therefore, care must be taken when using chemicals whose effects have not been previously documented in cats.

handling

The general case with animal work is that, unlike humans, animals do not cooperate with the proceedings and it is encumbant upon the users to learn to manage the animals. This is necessary to complete the project while minimizing the risk of injury to both the animals and the human handlers. Prior to handling animals, it is imperative that the process be carefully planned so that everything needed is available and the work can be quickly and calmly completed.

Information on cat handling is available elsewhere.[175,176] Cats are "borderline antisocial" in that they tend to interact with humans, and other cats, in a tenuous way that can disappear in a flash. Loss of the cat's tolerance leaves a blatantly belligerent or aggressive opponent.

Even minor handling can be stressful to cats.[24] In general, cats respond best to minimal restraint and hence it is best to allow the cat freedom at any time that it is feasible (Figure 7). They can often be gently "herded" around an exam table until restraint is required. If physical restraint is required by the procedure or for safety, then it is important to work quickly and maintain control and to release the cat as soon as possible.

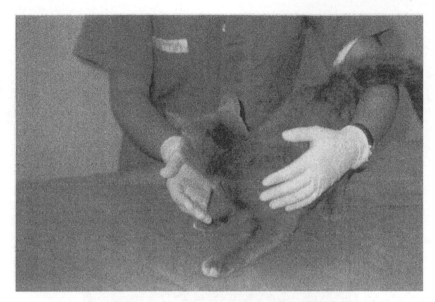

Fig. 7. Animal caretaker minimally restraining a cat.

Generally in this way, procedures are completely forgotten and cats quickly regain their composure.

Typical handling techniques are briefly described below:

Typical handling. Most cats can be picked up by grasping them lightly around the chest. They can also be handled by holding the loose skin over the shoulders while supporting their abdomen with the other hand.

The scruff. The loose skin of the dorsal shoulders and neck is referred to as the "scruff". Grasping this skin tends to make cats more tractable.[11] Cats can be lifted by the scruff alone but this is not usually done on a routine basis (Figure 8). The hold does not cause discomfort and it permits the handler to briefly avoid claws should they come into play.

Carrying. Cats should be carried by lightly holding the scruff while cradling the body between the handler's arm and body (Figure 9). It is often wise to restrain the forepaws using the hand of the arm supporting the cat.

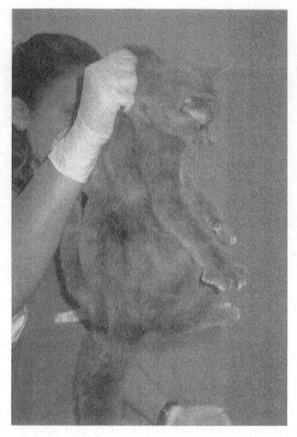

Fig. 8.   Cat held by the scruff. Note the protective mask, coveralls, and gloves worn by the handler.

Maximum manual restraint.   If a cat cannot be enticed to cooperate with a procedure, it can be fully restrained (Figure 10). This is done by taking a firm grip on the scruff, biasing your handhold towards the skin of the dorsal neck. Thumb and forefinger need to be towards the head. While lifting the cat with that hand, both hindlegs are grasped with the other hand. The index finger should be between the legs and the grasp should be just above the "hock" or heel joint. Thumb and index finger should be towards the paw. The cat is then laid on its side and extended. The restrainer's forearm should parallel the cat's back along the tabletop and extend

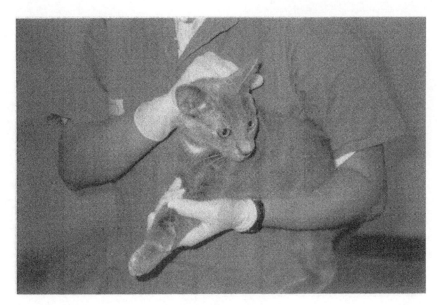

FIG. 9. Carrying a cat with one hand on the scruff and the other arm supporting the body. For better control of a rambunctious cat, the index finger can be passed between the "wrists" of the cat.

along the back to keep the cat from curling. This technique will completely control the cat and eliminate the possibility of injury to both the cat and those working with it. This technique requires two people as the restrainer is completely occupied with holding the cat and cannot do anything else.

One-handed technique.   Cats can be fully restrained with one hand if a second helper is not available (Figure 11). The technique frees up one hand for simple procedures like IM injections. It is done by lifting the cat by the scruff. To limit the cat's ability to turn, squirm and scratch, the restrainer grasps a hind paw and transfers it to a thumb–forefinger grasp of the hand holding the scruff. The scruff hold is maintained through finger–palm pressure. Strength is required for this technique as two separate holds are maintained by one hand and the cat must remain suspended in the air. This does not cause pain or injury to the cat but the hold should be used only for brief periods.

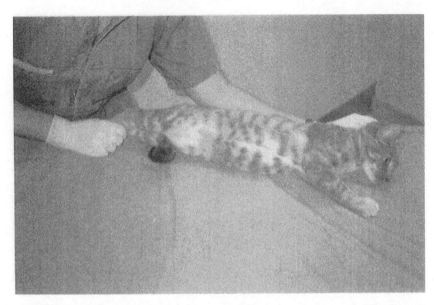

FIG. 10. Extending the cat and bracing it's back against the handler's arm. Some handlers prefer to have the index finger between the hind legs and to hold just above the "ankle" joint.

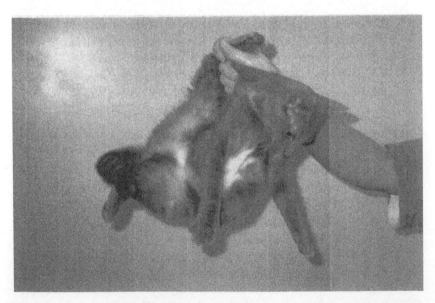

FIG. 11. One-handed restraint technique. Although not as desirable as having two people working together, this hold permits SQ and IM injections.

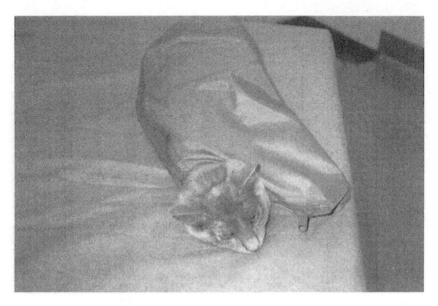

FIG. 12. A cat enclosed in a "cat bag."

handling devices

A number of devices are available for handling cats; these are briefly described:

Cat bags. A useful device is a "cat bag" (Figure 12). Cat bags remove the risk of scratches and cats tend to remain quite docile when enclosed. Cat bags are zippered or hook-and-loop closure bags into which cats are placed with their head remaining exposed. The bags generally can be opened very wide and unobtrusively closed up around a cat placed on them. They often have separate openings through which legs can be extracted for procedures. It is very difficult to get an angry cat into a cat bag so they should be brought into use before that happens. While cat bags effectively restrain claws, they do not protect from bites.

Muzzles. Muzzles are available for cats. These cover the face and eliminate the possibility of biting. Cat muzzles generally also cover the eyes so cats can be calmed (Figure 13). Again, they are impossible to get onto a belligerent cat.

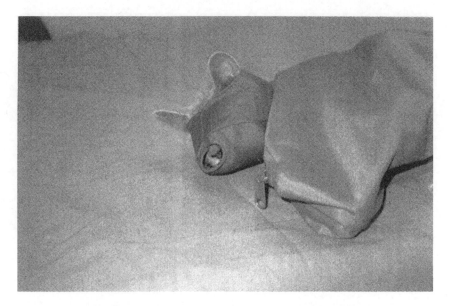

Fig. 13. Muzzle applied to a cat in a cat bag.

Towels, nets, and gloves. Towels, nets, and gloves can
be useful devices for controlling cats. Towels can be
thrown over the cat to reduce their ability to bite and
scratch by entangling them and inhibiting their ability
to see targets. Towels can be used to wrap up cats much
the same as a cat bag. Cats are very fast, and towel use
requires skill once the cat has resigned itself to fight.
Nets with handles allow the cat to be captured while
maintaining a safe distance; however, the cat can become
quite entangled and it may be difficult to get them out
(Figure 14). A wide variety of gloves can be useful. Light
leather gloves allow reasonably good feeling for the handler while providing some protection from injury. These
may be useful for handling the "borderline" cat that will
benefit from additional attention and socialization. Very
heavy-weight animal handling gloves are available as
well.

Snares and syringe poles. For extreme cases, snare and
syringe poles are available. A snare or rabies pole is a
long-handled device with a loop at one end (Figure 15).
The loop size can be controlled from the other end of the

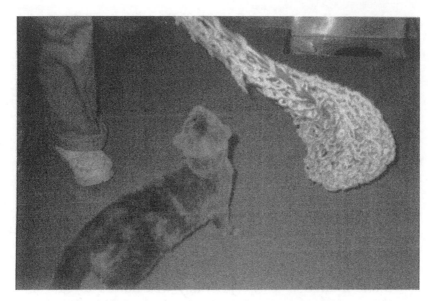

FIG. 14. Using a net to capture a loose cat.

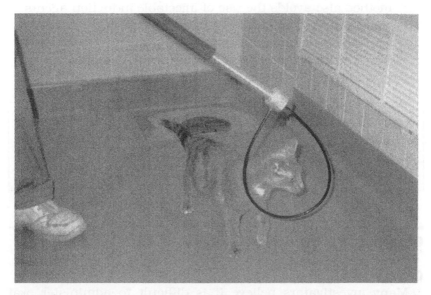

FIG. 15. Using a snare or rabies pole to capture a cat. Note that the potential for animal injury is high, so the snare must be specifically designed for the purpose and handled with care.

pole. The loop is placed around the cat's neck (or neck and foreleg) and tightened so it cannot be pulled off. The animal can then be held in place as it is injected with anesthetic or sedative drugs. The snare is not used to subdue the animal by choking it. Pole devices called syringe or punch poles are also available. These are long devices that accept a standard syringe on one end; the syringe plunger is activated from the other end of the pole. This allows injectable anesthetics to be administered while maintaining a safe distance from the animal.

Anesthetic induction boxes. Induction boxes are routinely used with cats. These are transparent plastic boxes with standard anesthesia machine ports. Cats are enclosed in them and the gases from an anesthesia machine are directed into the box. This method of anesthetic induction is exceptionally well suited to cats as they are "unrestrained" until anesthetized. Once the animal is anesthetized, it is removed from the box and intubated or maintained via a tight-fitting mask. This induction method also avoids the use of injectable induction agents that may need to be avoided for experimental reasons. Consideration must be made for protecting personnel from the anesthetic gas that will escape from the box as it is opened.

Note: Once cats are anesthetized, it is often advantageous to blunt the tips of the claws with standard small animal nail clippers. This dulls them enough to reduce injuries should the cat attempt to scratch in the future.

---

administering medicines and compounds

Oral

Many investigators believe it is difficult to administer oral compounds to cats. There are several methods for oral administration of compounds, including:

- **Incorporation of compound into the drinking water or food**. This rarely succeeds in cats as they are quite sensitive to tastes.

- **Administration by syringe**. For liquids that are readily consumed by cats, small volumes may be administered using a syringe by placing the tip of the syringe at the corner of the cat's mouth and slowly injecting the material.

- **Administration of pills**. With proper technique, it is actually very easy to "pill" a cat. This can be accomplished in a couple of seconds, it is safe, and done properly, the cat has no way to avoid the procedure. Being fast and hassle-free, cats accept it very well.

  1. The cat's head should be grasped from the top with fingers and thumb anchored against the bony ridges below the eyes. This should be done with the "non-dominant" hand (right-hander's left hand).

  2. The cat's head is turned so that the nose tip points toward the ceiling, straightening the neck (Figure 16). This makes it difficult for the cat to keep it's mouth shut and places the hand away from the forepaws.

  3. The pill should be held between the thumb and forefinger of the dominant hand while the middle finger pulls the mouth open by the incisor teeth (Figure 17).

  4. The tongue will be firmly curled, closing off the pharynx. While holding the mouth open, drop the pill in the center of the mouth near where the tongue is pressed against the roof of the mouth and push it over the tongue with the index finger.

  5. Immediately let the cat loose, the pill has been swallowed.

- **Gavage.** Liquids can be administered by gavage. This is necessary for liquids whose taste is objectionable. This is also useful for delivering compounds when the amount given must be precise. These techniques can also be used

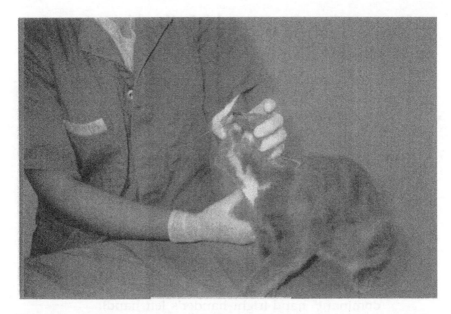

FIG. 16. Restraining the head and tipping the nose upwards in preparation for opening the mouth.

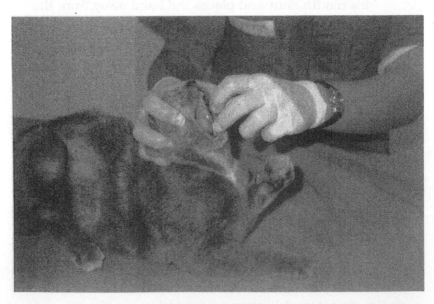

FIG. 17. Mouth held open as the pill is dropped into the back of the mouth.

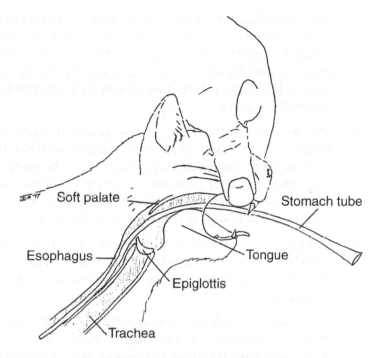

Soft palate

Stomach tube

Esophagus

Tongue

Epiglottis

Trachea

FIG. 18. Oral gavage of the cat.

for nutritional support of anorexic cats. Oral gavage is performed in the following manner (Figure 18):

1. Cats may need to be sedated for oral or nasal gavage.

2. The total length of tube to be inserted can be estimated as the length from the mouth to the last rib and should be marked on the tube before insertion is begun.

3. For unanesthetized cats, a speculum is placed in the mouth to prevent chewing of the tube. A small block of wood with a hole drilled in the middle to allow passage of the tube is sufficient.

4. The tube (usually an 8-French infant feeding tube) is lightly lubricated with petroleum jelly. For a nasogastric tube, 4 to 5 drops of 0.5% proparacaine should be instilled in the nostril.

5. The tube is passed through the speculum and back to the pharynx. Nasogastic tubes are passed through the ventral part of the nasal cavity. The head is maintained in the normal attitude; if the nose is lifted, the tube is more likely to inadvertently enter the trachea.

6. The location of the tube in the stomach must be confirmed to avoid accidental administration of compound to the respiratory tract. The tube should be examined for air passage as the cat breaths. One to 2 mLs of sterile water should be instilled as this will induce a cough if the tube is in the trachea.

7. Compound is slowly administered by a syringe attached to the stomach tube. Volumes of approximately 50 mL/kg per dosing do not appear to cause discomfort in cats.[40]

8. After administration, rinse any residual compound into the stomach by injecting a small volume of water and kink the tube to prevent flow of residual material into the respiratory tree as it passes through the pharynx.

- **Repeated Gavage**. For repeated administration, surgical placement of a pharygostomy tube should be considered. Under anesthesia, an oral feeding tube is passed and then the exterior end is exited through the pharynx behind the jaw. Long-term use of placed nasogastric tubes has also been successful.[177]

Parenteral

Most veterinary medications and anesthetics are administered to cats directly into the body (i.e., parenteral administration). Intravascular, intramuscular, and subcutaneous routes are commonly used and intradermal injections are sometimes done.

intravascular (IV)

Intravascular administration of compounds results in quick delivery to target tissues. Unless specifically required by experimental protocol, substances given intravascularly should be administered slowly, so that the consequences of an unexpected adverse reaction can be minimized. Blood samples may be collected from the same sites and by the same methods as those used for compound administration. The following points for intravascular administration and sampling should be considered:

- **Common sites** The most common site is the cephalic vein that runs along the forward surface of the lower forelimb. The medial saphenous vein of the lower hindlimb and the external jugular vein of the neck are used to a lesser extent.

➤ Administration Technique

Liquid compounds may be administered by needle and syringe. The technique is as follows:

1. Accurate venipuncture requires an understanding of the anatomy involved and practice. Working conditions must be optimized to improve the chances of the procedure being successful. Local anesthesia with a topical cream can be used.[178]

2. The cat must be adequately restrained. As cats prefer to "avoid interaction", some experienced handlers will place the cat on a slick table and grasp the paw. Since the cat cannot get effective traction, it will inadvertently immobilize itself as it pulls back from the handler (Figure 19). Cephalic venipuncture is often possible during the ensuing "stalemate." Minimal restraint is used and the loss of the paw and the needle stick are deemed acceptable since relative freedom is permitted for the rest of the cat. Restraint for cephalic venipuncture may also involve using an assistant to lean over the crouched body of a cat. One hand should control the head and the other helps holds the "venipuncture limb" from moving. Access to the jugular vein is best done by restraining the head and extending the neck while the other hand holds both forepaws (Figure 20). The forepaws and head are extended in a vertical line just beyond a table edge.[176]

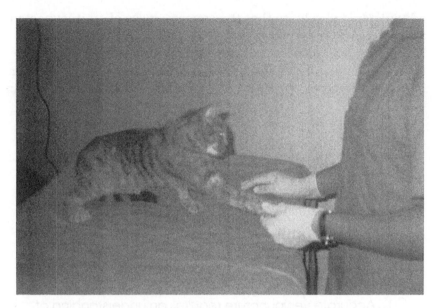

FIG. 19.   Grasping the paw for minimal restraint during veni-puncture can be successful with many cats.

3. The vessel must be located. Clipping the hair from the site greatly improves visibility of the vessel. Good lighting, a table of comfortable height, and a well-restrained cat are also important. Veins need to be occluded such that they fill with blood before venipuncture will be successful. This can be done by use of a tourniquet or finger pressure over the vessel between the work site and the heart.

4. Intravascular location is suggested by the presence of blood in the hub of the needle and the tip of the syringe shaft. This is further confirmed by pulling the syringe plunger back slightly to draw blood into the syringe. After confirming that the needle placement is correct, the tourniquet is released and the syringe plunger is slowing pressed. Formation of a bleb or blister around the vessel as compound is being injected indicates that the needle is not within the blood vessel.

5. Depending upon the viscosity of the compound, the smallest bore needle possible should be used. Generally, 20 to 26-gauge needles are used.

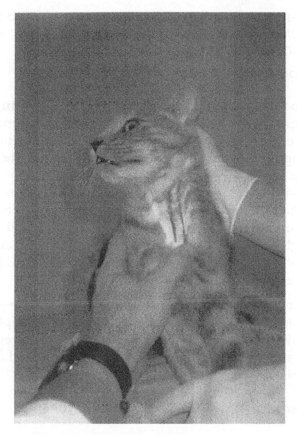

FIG. 20. Restraining a cat for jugular venipuncture. The cat's left jugular vein is outlined in black for demonstration purposes.

    6. Following injection, the needle is removed. Bleeding from the site is most effectively controlled by slight pressure. Excessively firm pressure excludes blood from the area; this can eliminate the hemostatic products required to stop blood leakage.

➤ *Sampling Technique*

The technique and sampling sites used are the same as those used for compound administration. Additional points to consider are:

    1. The syringe plunger cannot be pulled back too rapidly or the vessel will empty and collapse.

2. Generally, 5 to 6 mL of whole blood per kg body weight can be safely withdrawn from a healthy cat without ill effects. [179]

3. Typically, 22 or 23-gauge needles are used.

Chronic intravascular administration and sampling may be best performed through implanted catheters. The most commonly used vessels for long-term catheters are the jugular and femoral veins. Scrupulous **sterile technique** must be followed with long-term catheters as implant-related infection is very common.[178] Care must be taken when repeated blood samples are withdrawn to assure that the cat's ability to replace the blood is not exceeded. **Monitoring packed-cell volume** is advised but for planning purposes, roughly 0.5 to 0.6 mL per kg can be taken each 24 hours. [179]

Vascular access ports are available that allow repeated vascular access through an injection device implanted beneath the skin. Their use has recently been reported in cats.[180] The ports can also be used for repeated access to other internal structures.[181]

intramuscular (IM)

Sites.   The large muscles on the back of the rear legs or the musculature on the sides of the spinal column.

➤ Technique

1. Depending upon the viscosity of the compound, the smallest bore needle possible should be used. Generally, 22- to 26-gauge needles are useful for this application.

2. It is important that nerves and blood vessels be avoided when giving IM injections. The muscle mass should be firmly grasped and immobilized with one hand, while the other hand manipulates the syringe (Figure 21).

3. The needle is inserted through the skin and into the muscle.

4. The syringe plunger is gently pulled back to ensure that the needle is not within a blood vessel. If intravascular, a small amount of blood may appear in the syringe or the hub of the needle, and the needle should be repositioned.

5. In general, volumes no greater than 0.5 mL should be injected into a single IM site.

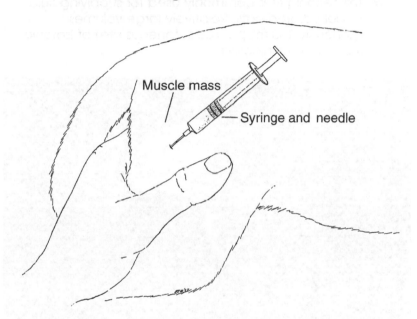

Fig. 21. Intramuscular injection into the large muscle bodies behind the femur.

subcutaneous (SC or SQ)

Site: dorsum (top) of the neck and back. Subcutaneous administration of compounds by needle and syringe is easily accomplished in cats due to the pliable skin and large subcutaneous space on the dorsum (top) of the neck and back.

➤ *Technique*

1. The smallest bore needle possible should be used depending upon the compound viscosity. Generally, 21-gauge or greater (smaller diameter) needles are useful.

2. A fold of skin on the neck or back is lifted (Figure 22).

3. The needle, with attached syringe, is inserted at a right angle to the skin fold. Once the skin has been penetrated, the skin should be released to minimize the possibility that the needle has exited the other side of the skin fold.

4. This technique is commonly used for supplying fluids to dehydrated cats. Relatively large volumes (generally 100 mL per subcutaneous site) of isotonic fluids can be injected.

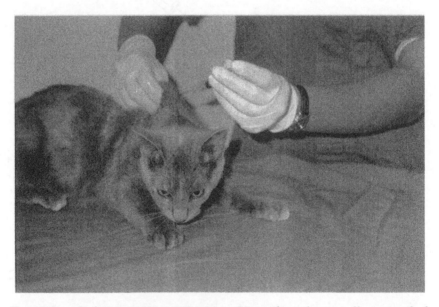

FIG. 22. Subcutaneous injection. Note that the needle is angled away from the head in case the cat jumps.

intradermal (id)

Intradermal injection is disposition of the material into the structure of the skin itself. It is not frequently used in cats.

Site. The skin of the trunk.

➤ *Technique*

1. The hair is shaved to adequately view the injection site.

2. A small bore needle (25- to 27-gauge), bevel side up, attached to a tuberculin syringe is used to penetrate into the dermis while the skin is held taut.

3. A small blister-like bleb forms within the skin on injection, confirming the intradermal location.

4. Small volumes of approximately 0.1 mL per site may be administered in this manner.

implantable osmotic pumps

Osmotic pumps are small, self-contained devices which are designed to deliver substances at a specified rate under the force of osmotic pressure. The pump can be implanted surgically into subcutaneous sites or into the abdominal cavity.

---

urine collection

The method of urine collection depends on the use of the sample and the tolerance for contamination with bacteria, feces, or other debris.[182] Urine should be collected in a clean, dry container and stored under refrigeration if the sample will not be used within several hours.

➤ *Technique*

1. **If sample contamination is not a significant concern**, urine can be sampled directly from the catbox. Absorbent litter must be replaced with material that will not absorb the sample (e.g., styrofoam packing "peanuts").

2. **Relatively pure** urine samples may be collected by **catheterization** of the urinary bladder. This is usually done under anesthesia. Careful use of sterile technique is important as the procedure can induce bladder infections. To perform this technique, a lubricated, sterile, 3- to 5-French flexible catheter is passed through the urethra and into the urinary bladder. In male cats, the penis must be elevated such that it is approximately parallel with the spinal column. This straightens the urethra so that the catheter may pass forward. In female cats, the urethral opening is located on the floor of the vagina.

An otoscope cone can be used to help visualize the urethral opening. Once the catheter has entered the urinary bladder, urine should flow through the catheter following gentle manual compression of the caudal abdominal region and under gentle aspiration pressure from an attached syringe.

3. **Relatively pure** urine samples may also be obtained by **cystocentesis**, a procedure in which a hypodermic needle attached to a syringe is passed through the abdominal wall and into the urinary bladder (Figure 23). Cats may be sedated but it may not be necessary. To perform cystocentesis, the cat is placed in lateral or dorsal recumbency and the caudal ventral abdomen prepared by clipping and thorough cleansing. Following localization and immobilization of the urinary bladder, a 22- to 23-gauge hypodermic needle is inserted through the skin and into the bladder. Urine can then be sampled under gentle aspiration pressure from an attached syringe.

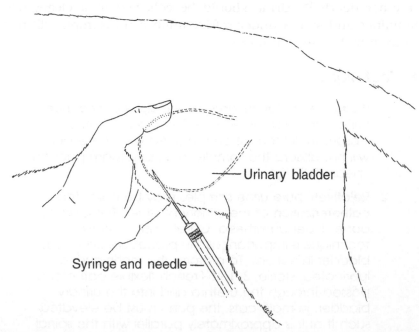

Urinary bladder

Syringe and needle

Fig. 23. Lateral recumbancy. Following surgical preparation of the site, urine may be collected by cystocentesis.

body temperature measurement

A standard measurement for assessing cat health is body temperature. Body temperature can be taken rectally using a small animal glass **rectal thermometer** with a small amount of lubricating jelly applied to the bulb. The thermometer is inserted 2 to 4 cm into the rectum and incubated for at least 3 minutes. Many cats object to the procedure. Alternatively, the body temperature may be measured from the tympanic membrane using an **infrared tympanic thermometer**.[113] This technique has the notable advantages of speed and acceptance by cats; however, tympanic membrane temperatures are typically lower than rectal temperatures and the technique is more sensitive to proper technique. The normal body temperature for cats, as measured by rectal thermometer, is 38.0 to 39.5°C (100.4° to 103.1°F) with circadian temperature swings of nearly 1°C.

endotracheal intubation

Endotracheal intubation is the preferred method of delivering inhalation anesthesia and cats have been used as a model for pediatric intubation.

➤ Technique

1. Short duration, surgical anesthesia is induced (see Table 9).

2. With the cat placed sternally, a helper grasps the skull and extends the head such that the nose points upward (but not directly vertical).

3. The anesthetist grasps the tongue with gauze and extends it out between the lower canine teeth and uses it to lower the jaw.

4. This generally affords excellent visibility of the larynx, although the soft palate may need to be elevated to release the epiglottis.

5. Laryngeal spasm in response to touch is not uncommon in cats. To reduce this tendency, the

larynx can be sprayed with 0.1 mL of 1 to 2% lidocaine from a 1 cc syringe

6. The endotracheal tube is inserted into the trachea at the start of inspiration (Figure 24).

7. The endotracheal tube recommended is 3 to 4 mm inside diameter.[152]

8. Proper placement of the tube is confirmed by expired breaths fogging the tube and by feeling the neck for the tube (which can be felt if it has entered the esophagus in error).

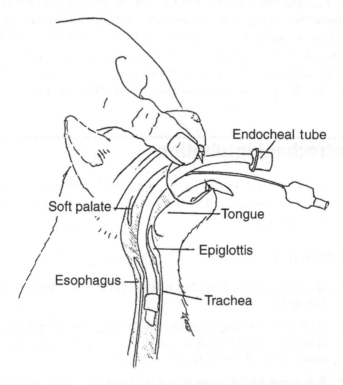

Endocheal tube

Soft palate

Tongue

Epiglottis

Esophagus

Trachea

FIG. 24. Endotracheal intubation of the cat.

necropsy

Many types of studies require the post-mortem examination of organs and tissues (necropsy). In addition, necropsy is frequently performed to diagnose disease problems.

➤ Equipment

Basic equipment needed to conduct a necropsy on a cat includes the following:

1. Latex or rubber gloves, lab coat, face mask, eye goggles, or other protective eye wear

2. A small metric ruler

3. Toothed and serrated tissue forceps

4. Scalpel blades and handles

5. Dissecting and small operating scissors

6. A probe

7. Bone-cutting forceps

8. Sterile swabs for bacteriological culture of tissues

9. Syringes (1 and 10 mL) with both large bore (18 gauge) and small bore (25 gauge) hypodermic needles

10. Fixative for preserving tissues for microscopic examination such as 10% neutral buffered formaline

11. Additional equipment may be useful and can be added to this basic kit

The necropsy is best performed in a dedicated necropsy room and on a surface that will facilitate drainage of blood and fluids. The area must be easily cleaned and sanitized. Stainless steel necropsy tables are optimal, and some are designed with downdraft air flow to draw hazardous agents and noxious odors away from personnel. If that type of equipment is unavailable, an area that is isolated from other animals, personnel areas, and feed and bedding storage could be used, provided that the area can be appropriately cleaned and sanitized following each use.

Formaldehyde, which is commonly used in diluted form as a tissue fixative, can cause allergic reactions and irritation of surfaces lined by mucous membranes.[183,184] In addition, formaldehyde is considered to be a human carcinogen.[185] For these reasons, steps to limit exposure of personnel to formaldehyde should be taken, including adequate ventilation of the necropsy and tissue processing areas.

Personnel conducting necropsies should wear a clean lab coat, latex or rubber gloves, a face mask, and protective eye wear. Although purpose-bred cats harbor few infectious agents that would pose a risk to humans, this equipment will further decrease exposure of personnel to airborne allergens and formaldehyde, as well as protect clothes from soiling with blood or other material.

Ideally, the cat should be necropsied immediately after death. Alternatively, carcasses may be stored for a short time (several hours) under refrigeration to delay tissue decomposition. Carcasses thus stored should be kept in refrigerators not used for storage of food for animals or personnel.

> **Note:** Freezing of carcasses can significantly interfere with meaningful necropsy.

Meaningful necropsy results depend upon a thorough familiarity with normal cat anatomy and experience with the changes that occur in tissues following death. General procedures for necropsy of a cat are as follows:

➤ *Necropsy Technique*

1. The cat is first examined externally for abnormalities such as discoloration, hair loss, wounds, masses, nasal or ocular discharge, and fecal or urine staining of the perineum. In addition, the oral cavity is examined.

2. The skin is incised along the ventral midline with the scalpel blade, beginning at the lower jaw and continuing along the midline caudally to the pubis.

3. Using the scalpel, the skin is then gently reflected laterally and the subcutaneous tissues and underlying musculature examined.

4. The abdominal wall is then incised and the abdominal cavity exposed.

5. The organs and peritoneal surfaces are examined for abnormal coloration, size, presence of masses, traumatic damage, or any other abnormal appearance. Depending on the time between death

and necropsy and the carcass storage conditions, the tissues may appear abnormal due to post-mortem autolysis, a natural process involving degradation of tissues after death and unrelated to disease processes.

6. The thoracic cavity is exposed by cutting the diaphragm and then clipping the ribs using the bone cutting forceps. The clipped portion of the rib cage is then lifted off and removed or reflected laterally.

7. The lungs, heart, and pleural surfaces are examined for abnormalities as for the abdominal cavity. The organs are removed for inspection by cutting the ventral floor of the oral cavity away from the jaw and cutting all attachments of trachea, lungs, and heart caudally to the diaphragm.

8. Abnormal fluids should be sampled for cytology and bacterial culture, and the volume and appearance of such fluids noted and recorded.

9. Other masses or abnormal tissues can be cultured using bacteriological culture swabs if infection is suspected.

10. Samples of tissues can be preserved in 10% neutral buffered formalin and saved for later histopathologic processing and evaluation. Samples should be no thicker than 1 cm to allow timely penetration by the fixative.

notes

resources

To provide the user of this handbook with information regarding sources of information, cats, equipment, and materials, examples of vendors and organizations are included in this chapter. The lists are not exhaustive, nor do they imply endorsement of one vendor over others. Rather, they provide a starting point for developing one's own list of resources.

organizations

A number of professional organizations exist which can serve as initial contacts for obtaining information regarding specific professional issues related to the care and use of laboratory cats. Membership in these organizations should be considered, since it allows the laboratory animal science professional to stay abreast of regulatory issues, improved procedures for the use of animals, management issues, and animal health issues. Relevant organizations include:

American Association for Laboratory Animal Science (AALAS), 70 Timber Creek Drive, Cordova, TN 38018 (Tel: 901-754-8620). AALAS serves a diverse professional group, ranging from principal investigators to animal care technicians to veterinarians. The journals, *Laboratory Animal Science* and

Contemporary Topics in Laboratory Animal Science are both published by AALAS and serve to communicate relevant information. AALAS sponsors a program for certification of laboratory animal science professionals at 3 levels: assistant laboratory animal technician (ALAT), laboratory animal technician (LAT), and laboratory animal technologist (LATG). The AALAS-affiliated Institute for Laboratory Animal Management (ILAM) is a program designed to provide state of the art training in laboratory animal facility management. In addition, the association sponsors an annual meeting and an internet site. Local groups have also organized into smaller branches.

The **Laboratory Animal Management Association (LAMA)** serves as a mechanism for information exchange between individuals charged with management responsibilities for laboratory animal facilities. In this regard, the association publishes the journal, *LAMA Review*, and a newsletter, *LAMA Lines*. The association also sponsors periodic meetings. The contact for LAMA changes annually with the elected president. The current contact for LAMA may be obtained from AALAS.

The **American Society of Laboratory Animal Practitioners (ASLAP)** is an association of veterinarians engaged in some aspect of laboratory animal medicine. The society publishes a newsletter to foster communication between members. In addition, the group sponsors annual meetings, generally in conjunction with annual meetings of AALAS and the American Veterinary Medical Association (AVMA). The contact for ASLAP changes annually with the elected president. Current contact information may be obtained from AALAS.

The **American College of Laboratory Animal Medicine (ACLAM)** is an association of laboratory animal veterinarians founded to encourage education, training, and research in laboratory animal medicine. ACLAM is recognized as a specialty of veterinary medicine by the AVMA and board certifies veterinarians as Diplomates in Laboratory Animal Medicine by means of examination, experience requirements, and publication requirements. The group sponsors the annual ACLAM Forum as well as sessions at the annual AALAS meeting. Contact is established through the Executive Director, who at the time of publication is Dr. Charles McPherson, 200 Summerwinds Drive, Cary, NC 27511.

The **International Council for Laboratory Animal Science (ICLAS)** was organized to promote and coordinate the development of laboratory animal science throughout the world. ICLAS sponsors international meetings every four years, with regional meetings held on a more frequent basis. The organization is composed of national, scientific, and union members. At the time of publication, the contact for ICLAS is Prof. Osmo Hanninen, Secretary General, Dept. of Physiology, University of Kuopio, P.O. Box 1627, SF-70211, Kuopio, Finland.

The **Institute of Laboratory Animal Resources (ILAR)** functions under the auspices of the National Research Council to develop and make available scientific and technical information on laboratory animals and other biologic resources. A number of useful publications are available from ILAR, including the *Guide for the Care and Use of Laboratory Animals* and the *ILAR Journal.* Contact with ILAR can be established at 2101 Constitution Avenue, NW, Washington, D.C. 20418 (Tel: 202-334-2590).

The **Association for Assessment and Accreditation of Laboratory Animal Care International, Inc. (AAALAC International)** is a nonprofit organization which provides a mechanism for peer evaluation of laboratory animal care programs. AAALAC accreditation is widely accepted as strong evidence of a quality research animal care and use program. Contact with AAALAC may be made through the Executive Director at 11300 Rockville Pike, Suite 1211, Rockville, MD 20852-3035 (Tel: 301-231-5353).

publications

A number of published materials are valuable as additional reference materials, including both books and periodicals.

Books

The following books may be worthwhile sources of additional information:

1. *Laboratory Animal Medicine,* by Fox, J. G., Cohen, B. J., and Loew, F. M., Eds., 1984. Academic Press, Orlando, FL 32887.

2. *Diseases and Management in the Multiple-Cat Environment,* by Pedersen, N. C., Ed., 1991. American Veterinary Publications, Inc., Goleta, CA 93117.

3. *Formulary for Laboratory Animals,* by C. T. Hawk and S. L. Leary, 1995. Iowa State University Press, Ames, IA 50014.

4. *Laboratory Animal Anesthesia,* 2nd ed., by P. A. Flecknell, 1996. Academic Press, Inc., Orlando, FL 32887.

5. *Handbook of Veterinary Anesthesia,* by W. W. Muir, J. A. E. Hubbell, R. T. Skarda, and R. M. Bednarski 1995. C.V. Mosby Co., 11830 Westline Industrial Drive, St. Louis, MO 63146.

6. *Restraint and Handling of Wild and Domestic Animals,* 2nd Edition, by Fowler, M. E., 1995. Iowa State University Press, Ames, IA.

7. *Laboratory Animal Management — Cats,* Committee on Cats of the Institute of Laboratory Animal Resources, National Academy of Sciences, Washington, D.C., 1978.

Periodicals

The following periodicals are excellent sources of current relevant information:

1. *Laboratory Animal Science.* Published by the American Association for Laboratory Animal Science. For contact information, see above listing for AALAS.

2. *Contemporary Topics in Laboratory Animal Science.* Published by the American Association for Laboratory Animal Science. For contact information, see above listing for AALAS.

3. *Laboratory Animals.* Published by Royal Society of Medicine Press, 1 Wimpole Street, London W1M 8AE, UK.

4. *Lab Animal.* Published by Nature Publishing Co., 345 Park Avenue South, NY 10010-1707.

5. *ILAR Journal.* Published by the Institute of Laboratory Animal Resources, National Research Council. For contact information, see above listing for ILAR.

electronic resources

Many on-line sources of information relevant to the care and use of laboratory animals, including cats, are available. These include:

1. **The American Association for Laboratory Animal Science (AALAS)** can be contacted for connection information. Some portions of the system are open to the general public and can be accessed at http://www.aalas.org/.

2. **Comparative Medicine Discussion List (COMPMED).** An electronic mailing list available through the internet, COMPMED is a valuable means to quickly tap into the expertise of laboratory animal science professionals around the world. Those interested in using this resource should AALAS for subscription information.

3. **The NETVET.** The Netvet is a vast collection of world wide web pages and links on all aspects of veterinary and animal matters. The site contains links to electronic versions of laws, regulations and policies. There are links to web pages of animal vendors, research institutions, scientific organizations and much more. The Netvet was conceived and developed by Dr. Ken Boschert of Washington University's Division of Comparative Medicine. The Netvet can be accessed at http://www.avma.org/.

4. **Network of Animal Health (NOAH).** NOAH is a commercial on-line service sponsored by the American Veterinary Medical Association. A number of forums cover a variety

of topics, some of which would be of interest to those charged with the care and use of laboratory cats. Additional information can be obtained from the American Veterinary Medical Association (1931 N. Meacham Rd., Suite 100, Schaumburg, IL; 1-800-248-2862; e-mail: 72662.3435@compuserve.com).

animal sources

Cats may be obtained from vendors of varying size and quality. Purchase of only specific pathogen-free (SPF) cats is strongly encouraged. Vendors should be asked to supply information regarding the health status of their cat colony for consideration prior to purchase. It is impractical to list all vendors here, however the following are examples of vendors which supply cats:

1. Cedar River Laboratories, P.O. Box 1462, Mason City, IA 50401 (Tel: 1-800-323-4858).

2. Harlan Sprague Dawley, Inc., P.O. Box 29176, Indianapolis, IN 46229 (Tel: 1-317-894-7521).

3. Kiser Lake Kennels, P.O. Box 541, St. Paris, OH 43072 (Tel: 1-937-362-3193).

4. Liberty Research, Inc., P.O. Box 107, Route 17C, Waverly, NY 14892 (Tel: 1-607-565-8131).

5. Martin Creek Kennels, P.O. Box 139, Williford, AR 72482 (Tel: 1-501-966-4345).

6. Summit Ridge Farms, R.D. #1, Box 131, Susquehanna, PA 18847 (Tel: 1-717-756-2656).

feed

Commercial cat food is readily available from local sources; however, most research facilities use feline diets produced specifically for the research environment.

1. Bio-Serv, Inc., P.O. Box 450, 8th & Harrison Streets, Frenchtown, NJ 08825 (Tel: 1-800-473-2155).

2. Harlan Teklad, P.O. Box 44220, Madison, WI 53744-4220 (Tel: 608-277-2066).

3. ICN Pharmaceuticals, Biomedical Research Products Division, 3300 Hyland Avenue, Costa Mesa, CA 92626 (Tel: 1-800-854-0530).

4. PMI/Purina Mills, Inc., 505 North 4th St., P.O. Box 548, Richmond, IN 47375 (Tel: 1-800-227-8941).

---

equipment

Sanitation
Several sources of disinfectants and other sanitation supplies are listed below:

1. Pharmacal Research Labs, Inc., P.O. Box 369, Naugatuck, CT 06770 (Tel: 1-800-243-5350).

2. BioSentry, Inc., 1481 Rock Mountain Blvd., Stone Mountain, GA 30083-9986 (Tel: 1-800-788-4246).

3. Calgon Vestal Contamination Control, P.O. Box 147, St. Louis, MO 63166-0147 (Tel: 1-800-582-6514).

4. Rochester Midland, Inc., 333 Hollenbeck St., P.O. Box 1515, Rochester, NY 14603-1515 (Tel: 1-800-836-1627).

Cages and Research and Veterinary Supplies
Several sources for pharmaceuticals, hypodermic needles, syringes, surgical equipment, bandages, and other related items are provided below. Pharmaceuticals should generally be ordered and used only under the direction of a licensed veterinarian. Cages should meet the size requirements as specified by relevant regulatory agencies. Stainless steel is preferable to galvanized steel.

TABLE 11. POSSIBLE SOURCES OF EQUIPMENT AND SUPPLIES

Item	Source
Cages and supplies	1,2,4,6,8,14,15,16,17,20,21,22
Veterinary and surgical supplies	4,7,10,11,12,13,14,18,24,25
Gas anesthesia equipment	5,11,13,23,24
Handling equipment	5,11,14,18
Syringes and needles	7,9,12,13,24,25
Vascular access equipment	5,11,18,19,
Osmotic pumps	3
Necropsy tools	9,11,13,15

contact information for cages, research, and veterinary supplies

1. Allentown Caging Equipment, Inc., P.O. Box 698, Allentown, NJ 08501-0698 (Tel: 609-259-7951 or 1-800-762-2243).

2. Alternative Design Manufacturing and Supply, Inc., 16396 Highway 412, Siloam Springs, AR 72761 (Tel: 1-800-320-2459).

3. Alza Corporation, 950 Page Mill Road, P.O. Box 10950, Palo Alto, CA 94303-0802 (Tel: 1-800-692-2990).

4. Ancare Corp., 2475 Charles Court, P.O. Box 661, North Bellmore, NY 11710 (Tel: 1-800-645-6379).

5. Braintree Scientific, Inc., P.O. Box 361, Braintree, MA 02184 (Tel: 617-843-2202).

6. Britz-Heidbrink, Inc., P.O. Box 1179, Wheatland, WY 82201-1179 (Tel: 307-322-4040).

7. Butler Co., Inc., 5000 Bradenton Ave., Dublin, OH 43017 (Tel: 1-800-225-7911).

8. Fenco Cage Products, 1188 Dorchester Avenue, Dorchester, MA 02125-1503 (Tel: 1-617-265-9000).

9. Fisher Scientific, Inc., 711 Forbes Ave., Pittsburgh, PA 15219-4785 (Tel: 1-800-766-7000).

10. Grams American Corporation, 2225 Dakota Drive, P.O. Box 192, Grafton, WI 53024-0192 (Tel: 1-800-366-1976).

11. Harvard Apparatus, 22 Pleasant St., South Natick, MA 01760 (Tel: 1-800-272-2775).

12. IDE Interstate, Inc., 1500 New Horizons Blvd., Amityville, NY 11701 (Tel: 1-800-666-8100).

13. J.A. Webster, Inc., 86 Leominster Road, Sterling, MA 01564 (Tel: 1-800-225-7911).

14. K.L.A.S.S., Inc., 4960 Aladen Exp., Suite 233, San Jose, CA 95118 (Tel: 408-266-1235).

15. Lab Products, Inc., 255 West Spring Valley Ave., P.O. Box 808, Maywood, NJ 07607 (Tel: 201-843-4600 or 1-800-526-0469).

16. Lenderking Caging Products, Inc., 1000 South Linwood Ave., Baltimore, MD 21224 (Tel: 410-276-2237).

17. Lock Solutions, Inc., P.O. Box 611, Kenilworth, NJ 07033 (Tel: 1-800-947-0304).

18. Lomir Biomedical, Inc., 99 East Main St., Malone, NY 12953 (Tel: 518-483-7697).

19. Pharmacia Deltec, Inc., St. Paul, MN 55112 (Tel: 1-800-433-5832).

20. Plas-Labs, Inc., 917 E. Chilson Street, Lansing, MI 48906 (Tel: 1-517-372-7177).

21. Snyder MFG. CO., 6228 South Troy Circle, Englewood, CO 80111-6422 (Tel: 1-303-706-9012).

22. Suburban Surgical Company, Inc., 275 Twelfth St., Wheeling, IL 60090 (Tel: 847-537-9320).

23. Vetamac, Inc., P.O. Box 178, Rossville, IN 46065 (Tel: 1-800-334-1583.

24. Viking Products, Inc., P.O. Box 2142, Medford Lakes, NJ 08055 (Tel: 609-953-0138).

25. Western Medical Supply, 117 E. Huntington Drive, Arcadia, CA 91006 (Tel: 1-800-242-4415).

notes

bibliography

1. Crawford, R. L., A review of the animal welfare report data 1973 through 1995, *Animal Welfare Information Center Newsletter*, 7 (2), 1-11, 1996.

2. Serpell, J. A., The domestication and history of the cat, in *The Domestic Cat: The Biology of its Behaviour*, Turner, C., Ed., Cambridge University Press, Cambridge, 1988, Chap. 11.

3. Wastlhuber, J., History of domestic cats and cat breeds, in *Feline Husbandry, Diseases and Management in the Multiple Cat Environment*, Pedersen, N. C., Ed., American Veterinary Publications, Inc., Goleta, CA, 1991, Chap. 1.

4. Leyhausen, P., The tame and the wild — another just-so-story, in *The Domestic Cat: The Biology of its Behaviour*, Turner, C., Ed., Cambridge University Press, Cambridge, 1988, Chap. 5.

5. Fitzgerald, B. M., Diets of domestic cats and their impact on prey populations, in *The Domestic Cat: The Biology of its Behaviour*, Turner, C., Ed., Cambridge University Press, Cambridge, 1988, Chap. 10.

6. Martin, P. and Bateson, P., Behavioural development in the cat, in *The Domestic Cat: The Biology of its Behaviour*, Turner, C., Ed., Cambridge University Press, Cambridge, 1988, Chap. 2.

7. Ilhan, M., Long, J. P., and Brody, M. J., Failure of heart rate response to cardioaccelerator nerve stimulation in Siamese cats, *Lab. Anim. Sci.*, 30(4 Pt 1), 657–660, 1980.

8. Kitch, H., Murray, R. E., and Cockrell, B. Y., Spina bifida, sacral dysgenesis and myelocoele, *Am. J. Pathol.*, 68(1), 203–206, 1972.

9. Robinson, R. and Pedersen, N. C., Normal genetics, genetic disorders, developmental anomalies and breeding programs,

in *Feline Husbandry: Diseases and Management in the Multiple Cat Environment*, Pedersen, N. C., Ed., American Veterinary Publications, Inc., Goleta, CA, 1991, Chap. 2.

10. Karsh, E. B. and Turner, D. C., The human-cat relationship, in *The Domestic Cat: The Biology of its Behaviour*, Turner, C., Ed., Cambridge University Press, Cambridge, 1988, Chap. 12.

11. Hart, B. L., and Pedersen, N. C., Behavior, in *Feline Husbandry: Diseases and Management in the Multiple Cat Environment*, Pedersen, N. C., Ed., American Veterinary Publications, Inc., Goleta, CA, 1991, Chap. 5.

12. Kerby, G. and Macdonald, D. W., Cat society and the consequences of colony size, in *The Domestic Cat: The Biology of its Behaviour*, Turner, C., Ed., Cambridge University Press, Cambridge, 1988, Chap. 6.

13. Turner, D. C. and Meister, O., Hunting behaviour of the domestic cat. in *The Domestic Cat: The Biology of its Behaviour*, Turner, C., Ed., Cambridge University Press, Cambridge, 1988, Chap. 9.

14. Rosenzweig, L. J., *Anatomy of the Cat: Text and Dissection Guide*, Wm C. Brown, Dubuque, IA. 1990.

15. Hart, B. L. and Pedersen, N. C., Behavior, in *Feline Husbandry: Diseases and Management in the Multiple Cat Environment*, Pedersen, N. C., Ed., American Veterinary Publications, Inc., Goleta, CA, 1991, Chap. 5., p 302.

16. Nuyttens, J. J. and Simoens, P. J., Morphologic study of the musculature of the third eyelid in the cat (*Felis catus*), *Lab. Anim. Sci.*, 45(5), 561–563,1995.

17. Ringler, D. H. and Peter, G. K., Dogs and cats as laboratory animals, in *Laboratory Animal Medicine*, Fox, J. G., Cohen, B. J., and Loew, F. M., Eds., Academic Press, Orlando, 1984, Chap. 9.

18. Hurni, H., and Rossbach, W., The laboratory cat, in *The UFAW Handbook on The Care and Management of Laboratory Animals*, 6th edition, Poole, T., Ed., Longman Scientific & Technical, Essex, 1987, Chap. 29.

19. Board on Agriculture and Renewable Resources, Subcommittee on Cat Nutrition, Committee on Animal Nutrition, *Nutrient Requirements of Cats*, revised edition, National Academy of Sciences, Washington, D.C., 1986.

20. Owens, J. M., *Radiographic Interpretation for the Small Animal Clinician*, Ralston Purina Company, St. Louis, 1982. p136.

21. Benjamin, M. M., *Outline of Veterinary Clinical Pathology*, 3rd edition, ISU Press, Ames, 1978, Part 2.

22. Buffington, C. A., Cook, N. E., Rogers, Q. R., and Morris, J. G., The role of diet in feline struvite urolithiasis syndrome, in *Nutrition of the Dog and Cat*, Burger, I. H., and Rivers, J. P.W., Eds., Cambridge University Press, Cambridge, 1989, Chap. 23.

23. Muir, W. W., Hubbell, J. A. E., and Skarda, R., *Handbook of Veterinary Anesthesia*, Mosby-Year Book, Inc., St. Louis, 1995.

24. Willemse, T., Vroom, M. W., Mol, J. A., and Rijnberk, A., Changes in plasma cortisol, corticotropin, and alpha-melanocyte-stimulating hormone concentrations in cats before and after physical restraint and intradermal testing, *Am. J. Vet. Res.*, 54 (1), 69–72, 1993.

25. de Lahunta, A., *Veterinary Neuropathy and Clinical Neurology*, W. B. Saunders, Philadelphia, 1977, 48.

26. Liddle, C. G., Putnam, J. P., Berman, E., Fisher, H., and Ostby, J., A comparison of chromium-51 and iron-59 for estimating erythrocyte survival in the cat, *Lab. Anim. Sci.*, 34(4), 365–370, 1984.

27. Benjamin, M. M., *Outline of Veterinary Clinical Pathology*, 3rd edition, ISU Press, Ames, 1978, Part 1.

28. Diggs, H. E., Ogden, B. E., and Haliburton, J. C., Vomiting and diarrhea in a cat colony, *Cont. Topics Lab. Anim. Sci.*, 34(1), 75–76, 1995.

29. Pedersen, N. C., Common infectious diseases of multiple-cat environments, in *Feline Husbandry: Diseases and Management in the Multiple-Cat Environment*, Pedersen, N. C.,

Ed., American Veterinary Publications, Inc., Goleta, CA, 1991, Chap. 4.

30. Hurni, H., Daylength and breeding in the domestic cat, *Lab. Anim.*, 15(3), 229–233, 1981.

31. Committee on the Care and Use of Laboratory Animals of the Institute of Laboratory Animal Resources, *Guide for the Care and Use of Laboratory Animals*, 7th edition, National Academy Press, Washington, D.C., 1996.

32. McCune, S., Enriching the environment of the laboratory cat, in *Environmental Enrichment Information Resources for Laboratory Animals: 1965–1995*, U.S. Department of Agriculture, Animal Welfare Information Center, Washington, D.C., 1995, p. 27.

33. CFR (Code of Federal Regulations), Title 9; Parts 1, 2, and 3 (Docket 89-130), *Federal Register*, Vol. 54, No. 168, August 31, 1989, and 9 CFR Part 3, (Docket No. 90-218), *Federal Register*, Vol. 56, No. 32, February 15, 1991.

34. Crouse, S. J., Atwill, E. R., Lagana, M., and Houpt, K. A., Soft surfaces: a factor in feline psychological well-being, *Cont. Topics Lab. Anim. Sci.*, 34(6), 94–97, 1995.

35. Baldwin, C. J., Peter, A. T., Bosu, W. T., and Dubielzig, R. R., The contraceptive effects of levonorgestrel in the domestic cat, *Lab. Anim. Sci.*, 44(3), 261–269, 1994.

36. Morris, J. G. and Rogers, Q. R., Comparative aspects of nutrition and metabolism of dogs and cats, in *Nutrition of the Dog and Cat*, Burger, I. H., and Rivers, J. P. W., Eds., Cambridge University Press, Cambridge, 1989, Chap. 5.

37. Board on Agriculture and Renewable Resources, Subcommittee on Cat Nutrition, Committee on Animal Nutrition, *Nutrient Requirements of Cats*, revised edition, National Academy of Sciences, Washington, D.C., 1986.

38. Kane, E., Feeding behaviour of the cat, in *Nutrition of the Dog and Cat*, Burger, I. H., and Rivers, J. P. W., Eds., Cambridge University Press, Cambridge, 1989, Chap. 9.

39. Martin, P. and Bateson, P., Behavioural development in the cat, in *The Domestic Cat: The Biology of its Behaviour*,

Turner, C., Ed., Cambridge University Press, Cambridge, 1988, Chap. 2.

40. Buffington, C. A., Nutrition and nutritional diseases, in *Feline Husbandry: Diseases and Management in the Multiple-Cat Environment*, Pedersen, N. C., Ed., American Veterinary Publications, Inc., Goleta, CA, 1991, Chap. 6.

41. Novotny, M. J., Hogan, P. M., and Flannigan, G., Echocardiographic evidence for myocardial failure induced by taurine deficiency in domestic cats. *Can. J. Vet. Res.*, 1994 Jan, 58(1), 6–12.

42. Fox, P. R., Trautwein, E. A., Hayes, K. C., Bond, B. R., Sisson, D. D., and Moise, N. S., Comparison of taurine, alpha-tocopherol, retinol, selenium, and total triglycerides and cholesterol concentrations in cats with cardiac disease and in healthy cats. *Am. J. Vet. Res.*, 1993 Apr, 54(4), 563–569.

43. Baggs, R. B., deLahunta, A., and Averill, D. R., Thiamine deficiency encephalopathy in a specific-pathogen-free cat colony, *Lab. Anim. Sci.*, 28(3), 323–326, 1978.

44. Davidson, M. G., Thiamin deficiency in a colony of cats, *Vet. Rec.*, 130(5), 94–97, 1992.

45 Buffington, C. A., Cook, N. E., Rogers, Q. R., and Morris, J. G., The role of diet in feline struvite urolithiasis syndrome, in *Nutrition of the Dog and Cat*, Burger, I. H., and Rivers, J. P. W., Eds., Cambridge University Press, Cambridge, 1989, Chap. 23.

46. Gaskell, C. J., The role of fluid in the feline urological syndrome, in *Nutrition of the Dog and Cat*, Burger, I. H., and Rivers, J. P. W., Eds., Cambridge University Press, Cambridge, 1989, Chap. 22.

47. Wardrip, C. L., Artwohl, J. E., and Bennett, B. T., A review of the role of temperature vs. time in an effective cage sanitization program, *Cont. Topics Lab. Anim. Sci.*, 33 (5), 66, 1994.

48. Ryan, L. J., Maina, C. V., Hopkins, R. E., and Carlow, C. K. S., Effectiveness of hand cleaning in sanitizing rabbit cages, *Cont. Topics Lab. Anim. Sci.*, 32 (6), 21, 1993.

49. Goodrowe, K. L., Howard, J. G., Schmidt, P. M., and Wildt, D. E., Reproductive biology of the domestic cat with special reference to endocrinology, sperm function, and *in vitro* fertilization, *J. Reprod. Fert. Suppl.,* 39, 73–90, 1989.

50. Tsutsui, T. and Stabenfeldt, G. H., Biology of ovarian cycles, pregnancy and pseudopregnancy in the domestic cat, *J. Reprod. Fert. Suppl.,* 47, 29–35, 1993.

51. Michel, C., Induction of estrus in cats by photoperiodic manipulations and social stimuli, *Lab. Anim.,* 27(3), 278–280, 1993.

52. Lawler, D. F., Johnston, S. D., Hegstad, R. L., Keltner, D. G., and Owens, S. F., Ovulation without cervical stimulation in domestic cats, *J. Reprod. Fert. Suppl.,* 47, 57–61, 1993.

53. Leyva, H., Madley, T., and Stabenfeldt, G. H., Effect of light manipulation on ovarian activity and melatonin and prolactin secretion in the domestic cat, *J. Reprod. Fert. Suppl.,* 39, 125–133, 1989.

54. Chakraborty, P. K., Wildt, D. E., and Seager, S. W., Serum luteinizing hormone and ovulatory response to luteinizing hormone-releasing hormone in the estrous and anestrous domestic cat, *Lab. Anim. Sci.,* 29(3), 338–344, 1979.

55. Wildt, D. E., Kinney, G. M., and Seager, S. W., Gonadotropin induced reproductive cyclicity in the domestic cat. *Lab. Anim. Sci.,* 28(3), 301–307, 1978.

56. Graham, L. H., Raeside, J. I., Goodrowe, K. L., and Liptrap, R. M., Measurements of faecal estradiol and progesterone in non-pregnant and pregnant domestic and exotic cats, *J. Reprod. Fert. Suppl.,* 47, 119–120, 1993.

57. Natoli, E., and DeVito, E., The mating system of feral cats living in a group, in *The Domestic Cat: The Biology of its Behaviour,* Turner, C., Ed., Cambridge University Press, Cambridge, 1988, Chap. 8.

58. Stubenfeldt, G. H., and Pedersen, N. C., Reproduction and reproductive disorders, in *Feline Husbandry: Diseases and Management in the Multiple Cat Environment,* Pedersen,

N. C., Ed., American Veterinary Publications, Inc., Goleta, CA, 1991, Chap. 3.

59. Munday, H. S., and Davidson, H. P. B., Normal gestation lengths in the domestic shorthair cat (*Felis domesticus*), *J. Reprod. Fert. Suppl.*, 47, 559, 1993.

60. Verstegen, J. P., Silva, L. D. M., Onclin, K., and Donnay, I., Echocardiographic study, of the heart rate in dog and cat fetuses *in utero*, *J. Reprod. Fert. Suppl.*, 47, 176–180, 1993.

61. Loveridge, G. G. and Rivers, J. P. W., Bodyweight changes and energy intakes of cats during pregnancy and lactation, in *Nutrition of the Dog and Cat*, Burger, I. H., Rivers, J. P.W., Eds., Cambridge University Press, Cambridge, 1989, Chap. 7.

62. Dieter, J. A., Stewart, D. R., Hoggarty, M. A., Stabenfeldt G. H., and Laskey, B. L., Pregnancy failure in cats associated with long-term taurine insufficiency, *J. Reprod. Fert. Suppl.*, 47, 457–463, 1993.

63. Olovson, S. G., Diet and breeding performance in cats, *Lab. Anim.*, 20(3), 221–230, 1986.

64. Pope, C. E., Keller, G. L., and Dresser, B. L., *In vitro* fertilization in domestic and nondomestic cats including sequences of early nuclear events, development *in vitro*, cryopreservation, and successful intra- and interspecies embryo transfer, *J. Reprod. Fert. Suppl.*, 47, 189–201, 1993.

65. Swanson, W. F. and Godke, R. A., Transcervical embryo transfer in the domestic cat, *Lab. Anim. Sci.*, 44(3), 288–291, 1994.

66. Gunn-Moore, D. A. and Thrusfield, M.V., Feline dystocia: prevalence, and association with cranial conformation and breed, *Vet. Rec.*, 136(14), 350–353, 1995.

67. Remillard, R. L., Pickett, J. P., Thatcher, C. D., and Davenport, D. J., Comparison of kittens fed queen's milk with those fed milk replacers, *Am. J. Vet. Res.*, 54(6), 901–907, 1993.

68. Martin, P. and Bateson, P., Behavioural development in the cat, in *The Domestic Cat: The Biology of its Behaviour*, Turner, C., Ed., Cambridge University Press, Cambridge, 1988, Chap. 2.

69. Hurni, H. and Rossbach, W., The laboratory cat, in *The UFAW Handbook on The Care and Management of Laboratory Animals*, 6th edition, Poole, T., Ed., Longman Scientific & Technical, Essex, 1987, Chap. 29.

70. Animal Welfare Act, United States P.L. 89-544, 1966; P.L. 91-579, 1970; P.L. 94-279, 1976; and P.L. 99-198, 1985 (The Food Security Act).

71. Health Research Extension Act, United States P.L. 99-158, 1985.

72. Office of Protection from Research Risk, *Public Health Service Policy on Humane Care and Use of Laboratory Animals*, 1986.

73. Box, P. G., Criteria for producing high quality animals for research, *Lab. Anim. Sci.*, 26(2 Pt 2), 334–338, 1976.

74. Fletcher, A. M., Hoskins, J. D., and Elkins, A. D., Germ-free technique for the rearing of kittens: a research tool, *Cornell Vet.*, 81(4), 365–378, 1991.

75. Hickman, M. A., Reubel, G. H., Hoffman, D. E., Morris, J. G., Rogers, Q. R., and Pedersen, N. C., An epizootic of feline herpesvirus, type 1 in a large specific pathogen-free cat colony and attempts to eradicate the infection by identification and culling of carriers, *Lab. Anim.*, 28(4), 320–329, 1994.

76. Stark, D. M., Hardy, W. D., and Angstadt, R., Prevalence of feline leukemia virus infection in random source laboratory cats. *Lab. Anim. Sci.*, 37(3), 317–319, 1987.

77. Palumbo, N. E., Taylor, D., and Perri, S. F., Evaluation of fecal technics for the diagnosis of cat liver fluke infection, *Lab. Anim. Sci.*, 26(3), 490–493, 1976.

78. Meanger, J. D. and Marshall, R. B., Campylobacter jejuni infection within a laboratory animal production unit, *Lab. Anim.*, 23(2), 126–132, 1989.

79. Coutts, A. J., Dawson, S., Willoughby, K., and Gaskell, R. M., Isolation of feline respiratory viruses from clinically healthy cats at U.K. cat shows, *Vet. Rec.*, 135(23), 555–556, 1994.

80. Glennon, P. J., Cockburn, T., and Stark, D. M., Prevalence of feline immunodeficiency virus and feline leukemia virus infections in random-source cats, *Lab. Anim. Sci.*, 41(6), 545–547, 1991.

81. Bradley, R. E. and Peters, L. J., Mebendazole paste as an anthelmintic in random source research cats, *Lab. Anim. Sci.*, 32(5), 523–524, 1982.

82. Nolan, T. J. and Smith, G., Time series analysis of the prevalence of endoparasitic infections in cats and dogs presented to a veterinary teaching hospital, *Vet. Parasit.*, 59(2), 87–96, 1995.

83. Committee on the Care and Use of Laboratory Animals of the Institute of Laboratory Animal Resources, *Guide for the Care and Use of Laboratory Animals*, 7th edition, National Academy Press, Washington, D.C., 1996, pp. 14–18.

84. Lappin, M. R., Feline zoonotic diseases, *Veterinary Clinics of North America: Small Animal Practice*, 23(1), 57–78, 1993.

85. Kasting G., Revisiting medical surveillance in research facilities, *Lab Animal*, 25(4), 27–31, 1996.

86. Hurley J, Working safely with research animals: employee and employer responsibilities, in *Proceedings of the 4th National Symposium on Biosafety: Working Safely with Research Animals*, Richmond, J.Y., Ed., Atlanta, GA, January 27–31, 1996, pp. 127–130.

87. Bascom, R., Occupational health programs, in *Proceedings of the 4th National Symposium on Biosafety: Working Safely with Research Animals*, Richmond, J.Y., Ed., Atlanta, GA, January 27–31, 1996, pp. 137–144.

88. Bascom, R., Occupational health and safety program in a research animal facility, in *Proceedings of the 4th National Symposium on Biosafety: Working Safely with Research An-*

imals, Richmond, J.Y., Ed., Atlanta, GA, January 27–31, 1996, pp. 65–69.

89. August, J. R., Dog and cat bites, *J. Am. Vet. Med. Assoc.*, 193(11), 1394–1398, 1988.

90. Regnery, R. and Tappero, J., Unraveling mysteries associated with cat-scratch disease, bacillary angiomatosis, and related syndromes, *Emerging Infectious Diseases*, 1(1), 1995.

91. Maruyama, S., Nogami, S., Inoue, I., Namba, S., Asanome, K., and Katsube, Y., Isolation of *Bartonella henselae* from domestic cats in Japan, *J. Vet. Med. Sci.*, 58(1), 81–83, 1996.

92. Childs, J. E., Olson, J. G., Wolf, A., Cohen, N., Fakile, Y., Rooney, J. A., Bacellar, F., and Regnery, R. L., Prevalence of antibodies to *Rochalimaea* species (cat-scratch disease agent) in cats, *Vet. Rec.*, 136(20), 519–520, 1995.

93. Merchant, S. R., Zoonotic disease with cutaneous manifestations, Part II, *Compend. Contin. Educ. Pract. Vet.*, 12(4), 515–521, 1990.

94. DeBoer, D. J. and Moriello, K. A., Investigations of a killed dermatophyte cell-wall vaccine against infection with *Microsporum canis* in cats, *Res. Vet. Sci.*, 59(2), 110–113, 1995.

95. Merchant, S. R., Zoonotic disease with cutaneous manifestations, Part I, *Compend. Contin. Educ. Pract. Vet.*, 12(3), 371–377, 1990.

96. Dubey, J. P., Mattix, M. E., and Lipscomb, T. P., Lesions of neonatally induced toxoplasmosis in cats, *Vet. Pathol.*, 33(3), 290–295, 1996.

97. Frenkel, J. K., Transmission of toxoplasmosis and the role of immunity in limiting transmission and illness, *J. Am. Vet. Med. Assoc.*, 196(2), 233–240, 1990.

98. Dubey, J. P., Toxoplasmosis, *J. Am. Vet. Med. Assoc.*, 189(2), 166–170, 1986.

99. Frenkel, J. K., Toxoplasmosis in human beings, *J. Am. Vet. Med. Assoc.*, 196(2), 240–248, 1990.

100. Pakes, S. P. and Lai, W. C., Carbon immunoassay — a simple and rapid serodiagnostic test for feline toxoplasmosis, *Lab. Anim. Sci.*, 35(4), 370–372, 1985.

101. Marrie, T. J., Q fever pneumonia, *Seminars in Respiratory Infections*, 4(1), 47–55, 1989.

102. Langley, J. M., Marrie, T. J., Covert, A., Waag, D. M., and Williams, J. C., Poker players' pneumonia: an urban outbreak of Q fever following exposure to a parturient cat, *N. Eng. J. Med.*, 319(6), 354–356, 1988.

103. Behymer, D. and Riemann, H.P., *Coxiella burnetii* infection (Q fever), *J. Am. Vet. Med. Assoc.*, 194(6), 764–767, 1989.

104. Meanger, J. D. and Marshall, R. B., *Campylobacter jejuni* infection within a laboratory animal production unit, *Lab. Anim.*, 23(2), 126–132, 1989.

105. Taylor, N. S., Ellenberger, M. A., Wu, P. Y., and Fox, J. G., Diversity of serotypes of *Campylobacter jejuni* and *Campylobacter coli* isolated in laboratory animals, *Lab. Anim. Sci.*, 39(3), 219–221, 1989.

106. Williams, L. P., Campylobacteriosis, *J. Am. Vet. Med. Assoc.*, 193(1), 52–53, 1988.

107. Nolan, T. J. and Smith, G., Time series analysis of the prevalence of endoparasitic infections in cats and dogs presented to a veterinary teaching hospital, *Vet. Parasit.*, 59(2), 87–96, 1995.

108. Kasprzak, W. and Pawlowski, Z., Zoonotic aspects of giardiasis: a review, *Vet. Parasit.*, 32(2–3), 101–108, 1989.

109. Zumla, A., Lipscomb, G., Corbett, M., and McCarthy, M., Dysgonic fermenter-type 2: an emerging zoonosis. Report of two cases and review, *Q. J. Med*, 68(257), 741–752, 1988.

110. Fogelman, V., Fischman, H. R., Horman, J. T., and Grigor, J. K., Epidemiologic and clinical characteristics of rabies

in cats, *J. Am. Vet. Med. Assoc.*, 202(11), 1829–1833, 1993.

111. Counsell, C. M., Bond, J. F., Ohman, J. L. Jr., Greenstein, J. L., and Garman, R. D., Definition of the human T-cell epitopes of Fel d 1, the major allergen of the domestic cat, *J Allerg Clin Immun*, 98 (5 Pt 1), 884–894, 1996.

112. Hollander, A., Doekes, G., and Heederik, D., Cat and dog allergy and total IgE as risk factors of laboratory animal allergy, *J Allerg Clin Immun*, 98 (3), 545–554, 1996.

113. Martin, B. J., Tympanic infrared thermometry to determine feline body temperature, *Cont. Topics Lab. Anim. Sci.*, 34(3), 97–100, 1995.

114. Lulich, J. P. and Osborne, C. A., Overview of diagnosis of feline lower urinary tract disorders. *Veterinary Clinics of North America: Small Animal Practice*, 26(2), 339–352, 1996.

115. Glennon, P. J., Cockburn, T., and Stark, D. M., Prevalence of feline immunodeficiency virus and feline leukemia virus infections in random-source cats, *Lab. Anim. Sci.*, 41(6), 545–547, 1991.

116. Pedersen, N. C., Yamamoto, J. K., Ishida, T., and Hansen, H., Feline immunodeficiency virus infection, *Vet. Immuno. Immunopath.*, 21(1), 111–129, 1989.

117. Ueland, K. and Nesse, L. L., No evidence of vertical transmission of naturally acquired feline immunodeficiency virus infection, *Vet. Immuno. Immunopath.*, 33(4), 301–308, 1992.

118. Yamamoto, J. K., Sparger, E., Ho, E. W., Andersen, P. R., O'Connor, T. P., Mandell, C. P., Lowenstine, L., Munn, R., and Pedersen, N. C., Pathogenesis of experimentally induced feline immunodeficiency virus infection in cats, *Am. J. Vet. Res.*, 49(8), 1246–1258, 1988.

119. Weyant, R. S., Burris, J. A., Nichols, D. K., Woo, E., Kinsey, V. S., Bower, D. E., Bukowski, M. M., Weaver, R. E., and Moore, T. D., Epizootic feline pneumonia associated

with Centers for Disease Control group EF-4a bacteria, *Lab. Anim. Sci.*, 44(2), 180–183, 1994.

120. Nasisse, M. P., Guy, J. S., Stevens, J. B., English, R. V., and Davidson, M. G., Clinical and laboratory findings in chronic conjunctivitis in cats: 91 cases (1983–1991), *J. Am. Vet. Med. Assoc.*, 203(6), 834–837, 1993.

121. Waters, L., Hopper, C. D., Gruffydd-Jones, T. J., and Harbour, D. A., Chronic gingivitis in a colony of cats infected with feline immunodeficiency virus and feline calicivirus, *Vet. Res.*, 132(14), 340–342, 1993.

122. Shelton, G. H., Linenberger, M. L., Persik, M. T., and Abkowitz, J. L., Prospective hematologic and clinicopathologic study of asymptomatic cats with naturally acquired feline immunodeficiency virus infection. *J. Vet. Int. Med.*, 9(3), 133–140, 1995.

123. Hart, S. W. and Nolte, I., Hemostatic disorders in feline immunodeficiency virus-seropositive cats, *J. Vet. Int. Med.*, 8(5), 355–362, 1994.

124. Femenia, F., Crespeau, F., Fontaine, J. J., Boucheix, C., and Parodi, A. L., Early haematological and pathological abnormalities of pathogen-free cats experimentally infected with feline immunodeficiency virus (FIV), *Vet. Res.*, 25(6), 544–554, 1994.

125. American Association of Feline Practitioners/Academy of Feline Medicine, *Recommendations for Feline Immunodeficiency Virus Testing*, 6808 Academy Parkway East NE, Suite B-1, Albuquerque, NM, 1996.

126. American Association of Feline Practitioners/Academy of Feline Medicine, *Recommendations for Feline Leukemia Virus Testing*, 6808 Academy Parkway East NE, Suite B-1, Albuquerque, NM, 1996.

127. Moriello, K. A. and DeBoer, D. J., Efficacy of griseofulvin and itraconazole in the treatment of experimentally induced dermatophytosis in cats, *J. Am. Vet. Med. Assoc.*, 207(4), 439–444, 1995.

128. DeBoer, D. J. and Moriello, K. A., Inability of two topical treatments to influence the course of experimentally induced dermatophytosis in cats, *J. Am. Vet. Med. Assoc.*, 207(1), 52–57, 1995.

129. Randolph, J. F., Moise, N. S., Scarlett, J. M., Shin, S. J., Blue, J. T., and Corbett, J. R., Prevalence of mycoplasmal and ureaplasmal recovery from tracheobronchial lavages and of mycoplasmal recovery from pharyngeal swab specimens in cats with or without pulmonary disease, *Am. J. Vet. Res.*, 54(6), 897–900, 1993.

130. Yagami, K., Furukawa, T., and Fukui, M., Serologic and virologic surveys on feline herpesvirus and feline calicivirus infections in cats for experimental use, *Jikken Dobutsu. Experimental Animals*, 34(3), 241–248, 1985 .

131. Hickman, M. A., Reubel, G. H., Hoffman, D. E., Morris, J. G., Rogers, Q. R., and Pedersen, N. C., An epizootic of feline herpesvirus, type 1 in a large specific pathogen-free cat colony and attempts to eradicate the infection by identification and culling of carriers, *Lab. Anim.*, 28(4), 320–329, 1994.

132. Nasisse, M. P., English, R. V., Tompkins, M. B., Guy, J. S., and Sussman, W., Immunologic, histologic, and virologic features of herpesvirus-induced stromal keratitis in cats, *Am. J. Vet. Res.*, 56(1), 51–55, 1995.

133. Stiles, J., Treatment of cats with ocular disease attributable to herpesvirus infection: 17 cases (1983–1993), *J. Am. Vet. Med. Assoc.*, 207(5), 599–603, 1995.

134. Evermann, J. F., Henry, C. J., and Marks, S. L., Feline infectious peritonitis, *J. Am. Vet. Med. Assoc.*, 206 (8), 1130–1134, 1995.

135. Olsen, C. W., A review of feline infectious peritonitis virus: molecular biology, immunopathogenesis, clinical aspects, and vaccination, *Vet. Microbiol.*, 36(1–2), 1–37, 1993.

136. Pedersen, N. C., Virologic and immunologic aspects of feline infectious peritonitis virus infection, *Adv. Exp. Med. Biol.*, 218, 529–550, 1987.

137. Martinez, M. L. and Weiss, R. C., Detection of feline infectious peritonitis virus infection in cell cultures and peripheral blood mononuclear leukocytes of experimentally infected cats using a biotinylated cDNA probe, *Vet. Microbiol.*, 34(3), 259–271, 1993.

138. Harvey, C. J., Lopez, J. W., and Henrick, M. J., An uncommon intestinal manifestation of feline infectious peritonitis: 26 cases (1986–1993), *J. Am. Vet. Med. Assoc.*, 209 (6), 1117–1120, 1996.

139. Biourge, V., Pion P., Lewis, J., Morris, J. G., and Rogers, Q. R., Spontaneous occurrence of hepatic lipidosis in a group of laboratory cats, *J. Vet. Int. Med.*, 7(3), 194–197, 1993.

140. Dimski, D. S., and Taboada, J., Feline idiopathic hepatic lipidosis, *Veterinary Clinics of North America: Small Animal Practice*, 25(2), 357–373, 1995.

141. Hawk, C. T. and Leary, S. L., *Formulary for Laboratory Animals*, Iowa State University Press, Ames, 1995.

142. Bradley, R. E. and Peters, L. J., Mebendazole paste as an anthelmintic in random source research cats, *Lab. Anim. Sci.*, 32(5), 523–524, 1982.

143. Kinsell, R. and Noyer, C. L., *Formulary*, Purdue University School of Veterinary Medicine, 1984.

144. Spoo, J. W. and Riviere, J. E., Chloramphenicol, macrolides, lincosamides, fluoroquinolones, and miscellaneous antibiotics, in *Veterinary Pharmacology and Therapeutics*, 7th edition, Adams, H. R., Ed., Iowa State Press, Ames, 1995, Chap. 43.

145. Norsworthy, G. D., Providing nutritional support for anorectic cats, *Vet. Med.*, 86(6), 589–590, 592, 594, 596–597, 1991.

146. Jackson, M. W. and Vail, D. M., Nutritional management of cats with infectious disease, *Veterinary Clinics of North America. Small Animal Practice*, 23(1), 155–171, 1993.

147. Anesthesia and paralysis in experimental animals: report of a workshop held in Bethesda, Maryland, October 27,

1984. Organized by the Visual Sciences B Study Section, Division of Research Grants, National Institutes of Health. *Vis. Neuro.*, 1988, 1(4), 421–426.

148. Muir, W. W. and Hubbell, J. A. E., *Handbook of Veterinary Anesthesia*, 2nd edition, 1995, Mosby-Year Book, St. Louis.

149. Flecknell, P. A., *Laboratory Animal Anesthesia: An Introduction for Research Workers and Technicians*, Academic Press, San Diego, 1987.

150. Center, S. A., Elston, T. H., Rowland, P. H., Rosen, D. K., Reitz, B. L., Brunt J. E., Rodan, I., House, J., Bank, S., and Lynch, L. R., Fulminant hepatic failure associated with oral administration of diazepam in 11 cats. *J. Am. Vet. Med. Assoc.*, 209(3), 618–625, 1996.

151. McMurphy, R. M. and Hodgson, D. S., Cardiopulmonary effects of desflurane in cats, *Am. J. Vet. Res.*, 57(3), 367–370, 1996.

152. Flecknell, P. A., Anaesthesia of common laboratory animal species, in *Laboratory Animal Anesthesia*, 2nd edition, Academic Press, New York, 1996, Chap. 7.

153. Millar, T. J. and Vaegan Arora, A., Urethane as a sole general anaesthetic in cats used for electroretinogram studies. *Neuro. Let.*, 1989 Aug 14, 103(1), 108–112.

154. Morgan, D. W. and Legge, K., Clinical evaluation of propofol as an intravenous anaesthetic agent in cats and dogs. *Vet. Rec.*, 1989 Jan 14, 124(2), 31–33.

155. Verstegen, J., Fargetton, X., and Ectors, F., Medetomidine/ketamine anaesthesia in cats. *Acta Vet. Scand. Suppl.*, 1989, 85, 117–223.

156. Remedios, A. M. and Duke, T., Chronic epidural implantation of vascular access catheters in the cat lumbosacrum. *Lab. Anim. Sci.*, 1993 Jun, 43(3), 262–264.

157. Andress, J. L., Day, T. K., and Day, D., The effects of consecutive day propofol anesthesia on feline red blood cells, *Vet. Surg.*, 24(3), 277–282, 1995.

158. Smith, J. D., Allen, S. W., and Quandt, J. E., Indicators of postoperative pain in cats and correlation with clinical criteria, *Am. J. Vet. Res.*, 57, 1674–1678, 1996.

159. ILAR, *Recognition and Alleviation of Pain and Distress in Laboratory Animals*, National Academy Press, Washington, 1992.

160. Adams, H. R., *Veterinary Pharmacology and Therapeutics*, 7th edition, Iowa State Press, Ames, 1995.

161. Borchard, R. E., Barnes, C. D., and Eltherington, L. G., *Drug Dosages in Laboratory Animals: A Handbook*, Telford Press, Caldwell, NJ, 1990.

162. Gilman, A., *Goodman and Gilman's Pharmacological Basis of Therapeutics*, 8th edition, Pergamon Press, NY, 1990.

163. Brock, N., Treating moderate and severe pain in small animals, *Can. Vet. J.*, 1995 Oct, 36(10), 658–660.

164. Taylor, P. M., Winnard, J. G., Jefferies, R., and Lees, P., Flunixin in the cat: a pharmacodynamic, pharmacokinetic and toxicological study, *Br. Vet. J.*, 150(3), 253–262, 1994.

165. Sawyer, D. C. and Rech, R. H., Analgesia and behavioral effects of butorphanol, nalbuphine, and pentazocine in the cat. *J. Am. Ani. Hosp. Assoc.*, 23 (4), 438–446; 1987.

166. McCurnin, D. M. and Jones, R. L, Principles of surgical asepsis, in *Textbook of Small Animal Surgery*, Vol. 1, 2nd edition, Slatter, D. H., Ed., W. B. Saunders, Philadelphia, 1993, Chap. 10.

167. Berg, R. J., Sterilization, in *Textbook of Small Animal Surgery*, Vol. 1, 2nd edition, Slatter, D. H., Ed., W. B. Saunders, Philadephia, 1993, Chap. 11.

168. Wagner, S. D., Preparation of the surgical team, in *Textbook of Small Animal Surgery*, Vol. 1, 2nd edition, Slatter, D. H., Ed., W. B. Saunders, Philadelphia, 1993, Chap. 12.

169. Powers, D. L., Assessment and preparation of the surgical patient, in *Textbook of Small Animal Surgery*, Vol. 1, 2nd edition, Slatter, D. H., Ed., W. B. Saunders, Philadelphia, 1993, Chap. 13.

170. Hobson, H. P., Surgical facilities and equipment, in *Textbook of Small Animal Surgery*, Vol. 1, 2nd edition, Slatter, D. H., Ed., W. B. Saunders, Philadelphia, 1993, Chap. 14.

171. AVMA Panel on Euthanasia, 1993 Report of the AVMA panel on euthanasia, *J. Am. Vet. Med. Assoc.*, 202(2), 229, 1993.

172. Osweiler, G. D., and Grauer, G. F., Toxicology, in *Feline Husbandry: Diseases and Management in the Multiple Cat Environment*, Pedersen, N. C., Ed., American Veterinary Publications, Inc., Goleta, CA, 1991, Chap. 7.

173. Bauer, M. C., Weiss, D. J., and Perman, V., Hematological alterations in kittens induced by 6 and 12% dietary propylene glycol, *Vet. Human Tox.*, 34(2), 127–131, 1992.

174. Hatchell, D. L., Reiser, H. J., Bresnahan, J. F., and Whitworth, U. G., Resistance of cats to the diabetogenic effect of alloxan, *Lab. Anim. Sci.*, 36(1), 37–40, 1986.

175. Fowler, M. E., *Restraint and Handling of Wild and Domestic Animals*, 2nd edition, Iowa State University Press, Ames, IA. 1995.

176. Sonsthagen, T. F., *Restraint of Domestic Animals*, American Veterinary Publications, Inc., Goleta, CA, 1991.

177. Abood, S. K. and Buffington, C. A. T., Enteral feeding of dogs and cats: 51 cases (1989–1991), *J. Am. Vet. Med. Assoc.*, 201(4), 619–622, 1992.

178. Flecknell, P. A., Liles, J. H., and Williamson, H. A., The use lignocaine-prilocaine local anaesthetic cream for pain-free venepuncture in laboratory animals, *Lab. Anim.*, 24(2), 142–146, 1990.

179. Joint Working Group on Refinement, Removal of blood from laboratory mammals and birds, *Lab. Anim.*, 27, 1–22, 1993.

180. Webb, A. I., Bliss, J. M., and Herbst, L. H., Use of vascular access ports in the cat, *Lab. Anim. Sci.*, 45(1), 110–114, 1995.

181. Remedios, A. M. and Duke, T., Chronic epidural implantation of vascular access catheters in the cat lumbosacrum, *Lab. Anim. Sci.*, 43(3), 262–264, 1993.

182. Osborne, C. A. and Stevens, J. B., *Handbook of Canine and Feline Urinalysis*, Ralston Purina Company, St. Louis, 1981.

183. Misiak, P. M. and Miceli, J. N., Toxic effects of formaldehyde, *Lab. Manage.*, 24, 63, 1968.

184. Greenblatt, M., Swenberg, J., and Kang, H., Facts about formaldehyde, *Pathologist*, September, 648, 1983.

185. Formaldehyde Panel: Report of the Federal Panel on Formaldehyde, National Toxicology Program, Research Triangle Park, 1980.

index

AAALAC (Association for
Assessment and
Accreditation of Laboratory
Animal Care International,
Inc.), 31, 101
Abdominal palpation, 43
Abscesses, 46
Accreditation, 31
Acepromazine, 59, 65
Acetaminophen, sensitivity to, 72
Administration of drugs, 80–87
abbreviations used, 50
anesthesia, 59–61
by endotracheal intubation,
93–94
Albumin, 7
Alkaline phosphatase, 7
Allergies, 39–40
Alloxan, 72
Alpha chloralose, 65
Alpha-melanocyte stimulating
hormone, 7
ALT, 7
American Association for
Laboratory Animal Science,
99–100, 103
American College of Laboratory
Animal Medicine, 100–101
American Curl breed, 2
American Society of Laboratory
Animal Practitioners, 100
American Veterinary Medical
Association, 69, 104
Amoxicillin, 51
Amylase, 7
Analgesia, 66
Anatomy, 4–6
Anesthesia, 53–65
administration of, 59–61
choosing a regimen, 55–57
euthanasia by, 68–69

in handling, 80
inhalation, 60–61, 69
records, 64
recovery from, 63–64
suppliers, 106
types of, 54
Anesthetic induction boxes, 80
Animal Welfare Act, 9, 13, 22, 24,
29
Anorexia, 52
Antibiotics, 47, 48, 51
Arachidonate, 71
Arginine, 15, 71
Aromatic carboxylic acids,
sensitivity to, 72
Aseptic surgery. See Surgery
Aspartate aminotransferase, 7
Aspirin, 67, 72
Association for Assessment and
Accreditation of Laboratory
Animal Care International,
Inc. (AAALAC), 31, 101
Atropine, 58

Bacterial monitoring, 21
Balanced anesthesia, 54
Barbiturates, 69
Barrier-housed cats, 34, 35
Bartonella (Rochalimaea)
henselae, 38
Basophils, 8
Bedding, 13–14, 17
Behavior, 3–4, 12, 14
assessment of, 42
handling and, 72
mating, 26–27
pain and, 64
Bibliography, 109–127
Bilirubin, total, 7
Biohazards, 40
Biological parameters, 7

Birth weight, 28
Bite wounds, 37–38
Bladder, 44
Blood collection tubes, 41
Blood pressure, 8, 66
Blood urea nitrogen, 7
Blood volume, 8
Body temperature, 7, 43, 62, 93
Body weight, 7, 28
Books, reference, 102
Bordetella bronchiseptica, 48
Breeding, 26–28
Breeds, 2–3
Buprenorphine, 67
Butorphanol, 63, 67

Caffre wildcat, 2
Cage cards, 25
Cages, 9–12
  design complexities for
    enrichment, 14
  grouped, 11
  sanitation procedures, 18–20
  suppliers, 105–107
Calcium, 7
Campylobacter, 39
Campylobacter jejuni, 49
Capnocytophaga canimorsus, 39
Carbon dioxide, 69
Cardiovascular function, 3, 8, 62
Carriers, 22
Carrying, 73
Casein, intolerance to, 71
Cat bags, 77
Catheters, 50
  intravascular, 58
  for urine sampling, 91–92
Catnip, 3, 14
Cats
  barrier-housed, 34, 35
  historical background, 1–2
  number used in research, 1974
    and 1995, 1
  phylogeny, 1, 4–5
  quality of, 33–36
  as research models, 71–72
  sources, 33–35, 104
  specific pathogen-free, 34

Cat Scratch Disease, 38
Census records, 25
Central nervous system,
    monitoring during
    anesthesia, 61–62
Cephalexin, 51
Cerebrospinal fluid values, 8
Certification, 100
Cheyletiella blakei, 38
Chlamydia, 48
Chloride, 7
Chromosome number, 7
Claws, 2, 5
Clinical chemistry values, 7–8
Coloration, 2, 58
Commercial vendors, 34–35, 104
Comparative Medicine
    Discussion List, 103
COMPMED, 103
Conditioning, 35–36
Conjunctiva, 42
Controlled substances, 55
Corticotropin, 7
Cortisol, 7, 66
Coxiella burnettii, 38–39
Creatinine kinase, 7
Ctenocephalides felis, 38, 47
Cyclomate, intolerance to, 71
Cystocentesis, 92

Dehydration, 50, 52, 58, 90
Dentition, 6
Dermatophyte test media, 46
Dermatophytosis, 38, 46–47
Dexamethasone, 51
Dextrose, 52
Diabetes mellitus, 49, 72
Diarrhea, 49, 51
Diazepam, 59
Diet, 15–18, 45
Digitigrade stance, 5
Disease. *See* Antibiotics;
    Infections; Parasites
Disinfection, 19, 41, 53
Dissociative anesthesia, 54
Domestic short hair (DSH), 3
Dosages
  analgesics, 67

anesthesia, 58, 59, 65
  drugs, 51
  recovery drugs, 63
Doxapram, 51, 63
Drug receptor sites, 72
DSH (domestic short hair), 3
Dysgonic fermenter-type 2, 39

Ear mites, 47
Ears, 42
Effusive form, of FIP, 48–49
Electrodes, 50
Electronic resources, 103–104
Elizabethan collars, 68
Endotracheal intubation, 56, 61,
  93–94
Enrofloxacin, 51
Enteric diseases, 49
Environmental conditions, 12–13
  during quarantine process, 36
  during transportation, 23
Environmental enrichment, 4,
  13–15
Eosinophils, 8
EPA (U.S. Environmental
  Protection Agency), 30
Equipment
  necropsy, 95
  sanitation, 20
  suppliers of, 105–107
  veterinary, 41
Erythrocyte lifespan, 8
Estrus cycle, 26, 27, 28
Euthanasia, 68–69
Experimental biohazards, 40
Experimental methodology,
  71–97
Eyes, 6, 42, 62–63

FDA (U.S. Food and Drug
  Administration), 30
Feces, 42, 58
Feed, 15–17
  in anorexia treatment, 52
  consumption per day, weight,
    7, 15–16
  gastrointestinal tract transit
    time, 7

  to minimize urinary tract
    problems, 45
  presentation of, 16
  removal of, prior to anesthesia,
    57–58
  storage, 16–17
  suppliers, 105
  during transportation, 23
Feed bowls, 11
Feet, 5, 63
Feline Calcivirus, 48
Feline distemper, 49
Feline Enteric Coronavirus, 49
Feline Herpes Virus, 48
Feline Immunodeficiency Virus
  (FIV), 45, 46, 48–49
Feline Infectious Peritonitis (FIP),
  48–49
Feline Leukemia Virus (FeLV), 45,
  46, 48
Feline Panleukopenia Virus,
  49
Feline Urological Syndrome
  (FUS), 44–45
Felis sylvestris catus. See Cats
Felis sylvestris libyca, 2
FeLV (Feline Leukemia Virus), 45,
  46
FIP (Feline Infectious Peritonitis),
  48–49
FIV (Feline Immunodeficiency
  Virus), 45, 46
Fleas, 47
Flunixin meglumine, 67
Formaldehyde, 95
Formalin, 95, 97
Fungal infections, 38
FUS (Feline Urological
  Syndrome), 44–45

Gastrointestinal tract, transit
  time, 7
Gavage, 81–84
General anesthesia, 53, 54
Genitalia, 5
Gentamicin, 51
Gestation, 27, 28
Giardia, 39, 49

Globulin, 7
Gloves. *See* Protective equipment
Glucose, 7
Glycopyrrolate, 58
Good Laboratory Practices for Nonclinical Laboratory Studies, 30
Greater omentum, 6
Griseofulvin, 47, 51
Group housing, 12, 14–15
Guide for the Care and Use of Laboratory Animals, 30, 31, 101

Hair, 42, 66
Halothane, 61, 65
Handling
  devices, 77–80
  manual, 72–76
Health records, 22, 25
Health Research Extension Act of 1985, 30
Heart rate, 8, 62
Heating pads, 62
Hematological values, 8
Hemoglobin, 8
Hepatic metabolism
  disorders, 49
  pathways, 71, 72
Herpes, 48
Historical background, 1–2
Housing, 9–12, 14
Humidity of cat room, 13
Husbandry, 9–28
Hyperthyroidism, 49

IACUC. *See* Institutional Animal Care and Use Committee
Identification, 25
  of sex, 37, 42
  USDA, 22, 24
ID (intradermal administration), 90–91
Ileum, 6
Illumination, 12–13
IM (intramuscular administration), 59–60, 88–89

Implantable osmotic pumps, 91
Implant problems, 50
Infections
  abscesses, 46
  antibiotics, 48
  commercial vendors and, 34–35
  enteric diseases, 49
  fungal, 38
  with implants, 50
  post-surgery, 68
  respiratory, 47–48
  retroviral, 45–46
  treatment, 50–53
  viral, 48–49
Infrared tympanic thermometer, 92
Inhalation anesthesia, 60–61, 69
In-house breeding, 33
Inspections, 29
Institute of Laboratory Animal Resources, 101
Institutional Animal Care and Use Committee (IACUC), 31–32
  pain assessment, 64
  protocol number, 25
International Council for Laboratory Animal Science, 101
Intestinal parasites, 47
Intestinal zoonoses, 39
Intradermal administration (ID), 90–91
Intramuscular administration (IM)
  of anesthesia, 59–60
  of drugs, 88–89
Intraperitoneal administration (IP), 60
Intravascular administration (IV), 84–88
Intravascular catheters, 58
Intravenous administration (IV), 59
IP (intraperitoneal administration), 60

Isoflurane, 61, 65
Itraconazole, 47
Ivermectin, 47
IV (intravenous administration),
    59

Jejunum, 6
Jugular vein, 86, 87

Kaolin-pectin suspension, 51
Ketamine, 61, 65, 69
Ketoprofen, 67
Kidneys, 6
Kittens, 28

Laboratory Animal Bulletin Board
    System, 103
Laboratory Animal Management
    Association, 100
LDH, 7
Legs, 5, 74
Lesions, 38, 52–53
Life span, 7
Lighting, 12–13
Litter boxes, 10, 11, 14, 91
Litter size, 27–28
Local anesthesia, 54
Lymphocytes, 8

Magnesium ammonium
    phosphate, 44
Maine Coon breed, 2
Major surgery, 55
Management, 29–40, 57–59. *See
    also* Records
Manx breed, 2, 3
Masses/swelling, 42, 43, 46,
    97
Mating behavior, 26–27
Mebendazole, 51
Medetomidine, 67
Metabolic disorders, 49
Methemoglobin, 72
Microchips, 25
Microsporum canis, 38, 46
Midazolam, 59
Minor surgery, 55
Mites, 38, 47

Monitoring
    anesthesia, 61–63
    microbiological, 21
    packed-cell volume, 88
    during transportation, 23
Monocytes, 8
Morphine, 59, 67
Mouth, 42
Mucous membrane color,
    58
Muscles, 6, 62
Muzzles, 77–78
Mycoplasma, 48

Naloxone, 63
Nasal discharge, 42
National Institutes of Health
    (NIH), 30
Necropsy, 94–97, 106
Needles, 41
    for cystocentesis, 92
    for ID administration, 91
    for IM administration, 88
    for IV administration, 86
    for SQ administration, 89
    suppliers, 106
Nepeta cataria (catnip), 3, 14
Nets, 78
NETVET, 103–104
Network of Animal Health
    (NOAH), 104
Neural tube development, 3
Neuroleptanalgesia, 55
Neutrophils, 8
Niacin, 15, 16, 71
NIH (National Institutes of
    Health), 30
Nitrous oxide, 61
Noise level, 13
Noneffusive form, of FIP,
    48–49
Normative values, 6–8
Nursing, 11
Nutrition, 15–18, 45

Occupational health, 36–40, 61,
    95. *See also* Protective
    equipment

Office for Protection from
    Research Risks (OPRR), 30
One-handed technique, 75–76
Oral administration, 80–84
Organizations, 99–101
Osmotic pumps, 91, 106
Otodectes cynotis, 47
Otoscope, 92
Ovulation, 26
Oxymorphone, 67
Oxytocin, 51

Pain
    analgesia for, 66
    assessment of, 64
Parasites
    external, 38, 47
    internal, 47, 49, 51
    treatment in quarantine
        process, 36
Parenteral administration,
    84–91
Passive integrated transponders,
    25
Pasteurella multocida, 37, 46
Pathogens. *See* Antibiotics;
    Infections
Penicillin, 51
Penis, 5, 37
Pentazocine, 67
Pentobarbital, 64–65
Periodicals, 102–103
Personnel
    allergies of, 39–40
    disease prevention hygiene by,
        53
    occupational health, 36–40, 61,
        95
    protective equipment, 20, 40,
        74, 78, 96
    responsibility for work records,
        25
    surgical clothes, 67
    zoonotic diseases, 38–40
Phenolic compounds, sensitivity
    to, 72
Phenylbutazone, 67
PHS (Public Health Service), 30

Phylogeny, 1, 4–5
Physical examination, 35, 36,
    42–43, 57
Physiology, 4–6
Pills, administration of, 81, 82
Piperazine, 51
Plasma volume, 8
Platelets, 8
Play toys, 14
Postsurgical management,
    67–68
Potassium, 7
Pre-anesthesia evaluation, 57
Predatory behavior, 4
Prednisolone, 51
Preemptive analgesia, 65
Pregnancy, 27–28
Procaine penicillin G, 51
Propofol, 65
Propylene glycol, 72
Protective equipment, 20, 40, 74,
    78, 96
Protein, total, 7
Psychological factors. *See*
    Behavior; Environmental
    enrichment
Puberty, 26, 28
Publications, 101–103
Public Health Service (PHS),
    30
*Public Health Service Policy on
    Humane Care and Use of
    Laboratory Animals,* 30
Pulse oximetry, 63
Purring, 5

Q fever, 38–39
Quality control, for sanitation,
    20–21
Quarantine, 35–36
Queen, use of term, 1

Rabies, 39
Rabies pole, 79–80
Records, 23–25. *See also*
    Management
    anesthesia, 64
    for transportation, 22

Rectal thermometer, 92
Red blood cells, 8, 71, 72
References, 109–127
Reflexes, during anesthesia,
    62–63
*Regulations of the Animal Welfare
    Act,* 29
Regulatory agencies, 29–32
Reproductive cycle, 26, 27, 28
Resources, 99–107
Respiratory function, 8, 62, 64
Respiratory infections, 47–48
Restraint
    handling devices, 77–80
    for IV administration, 85–86
    manual, 74–75
Reticulocytes, 8
Retroviral diseases, 45–46
Ringer's solution, 41, 58
Ringworm, 38, 46–47
Rodac plates, 21
Rotavirus, 49
Russian Blue breed, 2

Saccharin, intolerance to, 71
Salmonella, 39, 49
Sampling techniques, 87–92
Sanitation, 18–21
    disease prevention through,
        53
    equipment suppliers, 105
Sanitation test tapes, 21
Scent glands, 3
Scottish Fold breed, 2
Scratch wounds, 37–38
Scruff, 73, 74
Sedation, 55
Sex determination, 37, 42
Shipping containers, 22–23
Shock, 51
Siamese breed, 2, 3
Skeleton, 6
"Skin-tent" test, 50, 52, 58
Snares, 78–79
Social behavior, 3–4, 12
Sodium, 7
Sodium chloride, 41, 58
Solitary housing, 14

Specific pathogen-free cats (SPF),
    34
Spleen, 6
Sporothrix schenckii, 38
Struvite uroliths, 44
Subcutaneous administration
    (SQ)
    of anesthesia, 60
    of drugs, 89–90
Surgery, 66–67. *See also*
    Anesthesia
    postsurgical management,
        67–68
    types of, 55
Surgical anesthesia, 54
Survival surgery, 55
Sutures, 68
Swelling. *See* Masses/swelling
Syringe poles, 78–80
Syringes, 41, 95, 106

Taurine, 15, 16, 71
Teats, 6
Teeth, 6
Temperature
    body, 7, 43, 57, 62, 93
    cat room, 12
    environment during
        transportation, 23
Terminal surgery, 55
Tetracycline, 51
Thermometers, 41, 93
Thiamine, 16
Thiamylal, 65
Thoracic cavity, 97
Tiletamine, 65
Tissue glue, 68
Tom, use of term, 1
Total bilirubin, 7
Total protein, 7
Towels for handling, 78
Toxoplasmosis gondii, 38
Toys, 14
Tranquilization, 55, 59
Transportation, 21–23
Treatment of disease,
    50–53
Tumors. *See* Masses/swelling

Ungual process, 5
Urethane, 65
Urethral obstruction, 44–45
Urinary bladder, 44
Urine, 7, 42
    Feline Urological Syndrome,
        44–45
    pH, 45
    sampling, 91–92
U.S. Department of Agriculture
    (USDA), 1, 29–30
    commercial vendor
        classification, 34
    records, 24, 64
U.S. Environmental Protection
    Agency (EPA), 30
U.S. Food and Drug
    Administration (FDA),
    30

Vaccinations, 36, 39, 48
Vascular access ports, 88
Ventilation, 13, 95

Veterinary care, 41–69
Vitamin A, 15, 16, 71
Vocalization, 64

Water, 18
    intake per day, 7, 18
    to minimize urinary tract
        problems, 45
    removal of, prior to anesthesia,
        57–58
    during transportation,
        23
Water bowls, 11, 42
Weight, 7, 28
White blood cells, 8
Work records, 25

Xylazine, 59, 65, 67, 69

Yohimbine, 63

Zolezepam, 65
Zoonotic diseases, 38–40

notes

notes

notes

notes

notes

notes

notes

notes

notes